A holistic guide to living with hepatitis and liver disease

HEALING HEPATITIS & LIVER DISEASE NATURALLY

How time tested natural medicines can start the healing process

Detoxification & liver gallbladder flush.Reduce the risk of hepatitis, C, Hepatitis B,liver cirrhosis and high blood cholesterol with alternative remedies

How to achieve sustained viral clearance with natural remedies

Dr Peter I. Oyakhire
OD NHD PhD FAAO

Also Includes the Liver Cleansing Diet and Cookbook

authorHOUSE®

AuthorHouse™
1663 Liberty Drive
Bloomington, IN 47403
www.authorhouse.com
Phone: 1-800-839-8640

First published by AuthorHouse   11/17/2010

ISBN: 978-1-4520-1034-2 (e)
ISBN: 978-1-4520-1033-5 (sc)

Library of Congress Control Number: 2010904899

Printed in the United States of America
Bloomington, Indiana

Contents

Liver disease and beyond-the good news

When optometrist, herbalist, and naturopath Dr. Peter Oyakhire wrote *Healing Hepatitis & Liver Disease Naturally*, he was in the midst of his own midlife change occasioned by series of crises that includes infectious hepatitis, cancer of the lymph nodes, and liver cirrhosis. The good news, according to Dr. Oyakhire, is that liver disease and cancer are adversities that lead him to venture into naturopathy and holistic health. It became an opportunity for rejuvenation and reinvention of life that can be channeled for new adventures. He encourages individuals with liver disease to explore supervised alternative remedies with conventional remedies as adjuncts.

When Dr. Peter Oyakhire empathizes with liver patients, he is not pretending he knows what they are going through. After being diagnosed with lymphoma, Peter started a chemotherapy regimen that was expected to last about five months. About three months into therapy, he suddenly went into coma and the doctors discovered he has chronic hepatitis B, liver failure, and end-stage liver cirrhosis with less than 10 percent of functional liver capacity left. With the diminution of his kidney and lung functions, he was put on maximum life support. This made it impossible for him to continue chemotherapy. After being admitted into the hospital for six months, the doctors gave up on him. He was sent home to die. With his back against the wall, he veered from the path of conventional medicine to a trail that led to a wide variety of alternatives that help restored his health. He had to get out of the box to get healed. In this book, Peter takes us with unwavering honesty from his adversities to his disease-free state. He leads us step by step through a wide range of natural medicines and modalities, entirely bypassing conventional allopathic medicine. And in this book there is no room for victimhood.

Along with providing a wide varieties of alternative modalities for the treatment and management of liver diseases, this leading expert on nutritional immunology is pointing out to people with liver diseases that to heal completely they need to tidy up their unfinished emotional business, change unproductive relationships and lifestyles that increase stress, and reclaim ones life so that it is fuelled by what is real and sustainable.

Dr Oyakhire believes we can learn a lot from crayons: Some may be sharp, others may be short, some may be tall, and are different sizes, but they all have to co-exist in the same box. He believes that a big tent can be formed that acts as an umbrella that benefits humanity when the best of alternative and conventional approaches to the management of liver disease are employed for the good of the patient. Unfortunately, this is not so at the moment. Many people will die needlessly of liver disease and Dr. Oyakhire recommends periodic screening for all adults. He says "No one is marked down by genetic predisposition to degenerative liver disease or chronic illness." He believes that proper diet, lifestyles change, exercise, and a good night's sleep can prevent disease and genetic predisposition to any degenerative disease. His nutritional advice for individuals with liver disease is well documented in the following chapters. Peter advocates detoxifications as pre-conditions for healing combined with a diet rich in fruits, vegetables, grains, legumes, complex carbohydrates, and low in meat. Dr. Oyakhire exemplifies somebody who combines the best of mainstay medical diagnosis with complimentary alternative remedies producing remarkable results. His ability to integrate orthodox medicine with holistic remedies helped reversed his condition.

Civilization has given us foods which are synthetically fertilized, sprayed for bugs, preserved for shelf life, and sweetened for flavor. The lifeless end-products are re-enriched with synthetic vitamins and minerals. As humans consume these foods, our organ systems become artificial and react to those chemicals by manifesting disease symptoms. Conventional medicine responds with more synthetic drugs to sustain our life. The human body works 24 hours a day replacing about 300 million dead cells every minute. The replacement is contingent on the quality of the raw material that it is being supplied exogenously from food sources. The standard American and Western diets supply the body with dead building blocks which favors the continuation of diseased cells, organs, and organisms. These approaches perpetuate disease conditions .When we replaced millet with processed wheat and consume food devoid of the needed building blocks, the blood borrows from the bones, saliva, and tissues to sustain the needed PH for survival. This leaves the organs and tissues acidic and oxygen deficient which sets the stage for degeneration. Two-time Nobel Laureate Linus Pauling corroborates this view when he indicated that our ability to manufacture vitamins was discarded at a time when our ancestors lived in close proximity to fruits and vegetables and did not need to produce them within themselves. With evolution, industrialization and modernization, they moved from fruit and vegetable habitats to more organized settlements and suffered great deficiencies. He believed these nutritional deficiencies coupled with modernized farming, inadequate supplementation, and aquaculture have led to the proliferation of deficiency diseases.

Dr Oyakhire believes that with right attitudes and proper nutritional and holistic support, everyone can rediscover how it feels to be well again. When it comes to nutrition, he advocates nutritious, dense whole foods, and generous use of supplements to address nutritional deficiencies. He encourages individuals with liver diseases to reactivate the anti-oxidation system to combat oxidative stress with liver- support herbs

McCaulay Bensen: Liver disease survivor

In Loving Memory of my brother Ifijeh Ayo Oyakhire

Acknowledgements:

I wish to thank my wife Valerie Oyakhire for her emotional and spiritual support. Her words of encouragements through the years have sustained me. She is a jewel of infinitesimal value. I would also like to thank my children Isuan, Izegboya and Ofuan for their emotional support. I would like to express my sincere thanks to my sister-in-laws Ms. Uche Ehimiaghe and Ms. Nkechi Onogwu who were always there to provide me with moral, physical and spiritual support and encouragement. I also wish to thank Pastor Mike Adebiyi and Dr. Omoh T. Ojior for their supplications on my behalf. I wish to express my sincere appreciation to Professor Olanrewaju Oriowo, my bosom friend and colleague for his keen guidance in the valleys and celebration at the hilltop. I am grateful to my elder brother John Oyakhire for his moral support. My sincere thanks go to Mrs. Monika Frazier-Cross for helping put the dots, comas and question marks where they belong.

Introduction

Live your lifetime with liver disease:
A death sentence – A life experience
After months of excruciating pains, palpitations, breathing difficulties, and night sweats, I began to notice loss of energy during the day and falling asleep at odd times. I also noticed remarkable enlargements in my neck and jaw areas, which made me look very robust and plump. These occurrences coincided with my yearly routine physical, so I promptly made these complaints to the doctor. I was referred to the hospital where a diagnosis of non-Hodgkin's lymphoma was confirmed. I started a chemotherapy regimen that was expected to last about five months. About three months into therapy, I suddenly went into a coma and the doctors discovered I had developed hepatitis B, liver failure, and end-stage liver cirrhosis with less than 10 percent functional liver capacity left. I became totally jaundiced and yellow like mustard. I was put on a ventilator and was incubated to secure the airway after suffering anoxic neurological damage. I had a cascade of chemical reactions that opened the gates for toxins hence my systemic liver, lung, and kidney collapse. If things were not done medically to reverse this trend, I would have ended up in a vegetative state in 8 – 10 minutes. I could neither talk nor blink, and was in catatonic state, with only the severely compromised brain ticking away. My algorithms were very erratic on the monitor. A tube was inserted to access my lungs to see if a miracle could happen as soon as I arrived in the hospital, because my airway had been compromised by the time I got there. I was artificially kept alive as my heart was still registering on the monitor, no matter how poor my algorithm was. I was dead and alive at the same time, expecting a miraculous comeback. I could not move or make any form of communication because of the tubes in my throat and through my nasal septum.

This situation made it impossible for me to continue chemotherapy. While I lingered in coma, my wife would dutifully show up at the hospital each morning at about 4 am dressed as if she was going to my homecoming. Often, she would not leave until after midnight. We consoled ourselves with the words of country singer Naomi Judd: *"Don't allow your pain to be a prison, broaden your horizons, and make your illness a prism through which you see a higher calling and a new beginning. It is important to step out in faith, pray for the answer instead of solving the problem, live beyond the immediate physical circumstances and strive to pray for hope."*

I was determined to figure out what else I could do to enhance the long-term effectiveness of these conventional treatments and fully recover physically, mentally, emotionally, and spiritually by identifying and changing various aspects of my lifestyle. The challenge that I accepted for myself was to see if I could put together alternative remedies, looking for the best ingredients that conventional oncology therapy had to offer, and complementing it with additional therapies from the uncharted world of "naturopathy." I wanted to try to "tweak my fate" by tipping the scales in my favor of both fighting the disease and achieving the optimal health possible. This book is borne out of my desire to turn my pain to purpose.

Through what others would call an adversity, I deem a blessing in disguise, even though I was left between a rock and a hard place. I was faced with only one choice—to research alternative avenues of healing. While sequestered in a hospital with a life-threatening illness for six months and coming in and out of coma with two code-blue episodes, I watched my 5 foot 5 inch frame wither to 90 pounds, with high viral load, and a cancer that had spread to my abdomen's peritoneal cavity, liver, lungs, kidney, heart, neck, and was moving into the brain. I was told I had metastatic non-Hodgkin lymphoma, which the doctors told me it was end stage.

Things got so stirred up inside my body that the cancer, cirrhosis, and hepatitis B were in a progressive state and there was really nothing left to do but to get my affairs in order. I became an orphaned patient, medically. Sick, tired, and painfully aware that we had hit the bottom, my wife and I turned to the only option left—God. We veered into alternative healing therapies to find healing.

With only a rudimentary knowledge of herbs, I began a frantic research process of testing herbal formulas, alternative lifestyles, and healing food combinations, using my body as the guinea pig. I read voraciously about herbal healing. Family friends helped me shop for herbs, and I began to formulate the many herbal combinations that would eventually save my life. I was amazed as I watched my body restore itself back to life and wholeness, with my viral loads becoming undetectable, the lymphoma that was the size of a grapefruit reduced to a non-pathological peanut size.

Studies show that all health and wellness traditions except western medicine offer detoxification and toxic waste management as a means of natural healing and avoiding illness. Using the principles of natural healing and detoxification, Dr. Alexis Carrel, a Nobel Prize winner kept chicken heart alive for 38 years. He believed that cells could live indefinitely and that the secret of life is to feed nutrients to cells and to saturate the cells with Oxygen. If you can't get nutrients into the cells and you don't remove the toxins, the cells will be poisoned by their own waste products.

Research show that disease is nothing more than the body responding to the wrong we have done to it. It is the body's attempt at keeping us alive in response to the wrongs we have inflicted on our bodies. If the body has the intelligence to produce a disease, it is capable of reversing the process to return to health once the cause is removed. The foundation of any disease state is "toxemia", i.e. progressive accumulation of metabolic and environmental wastes that the body fails to excrete through its normal elimination channels, storing them instead in the tissues. The body was not able effectively undergo detoxification because of "enervation", or the lack of vitality due to faulty metabolism.

In understanding the principles behind the principal supplements it this book, you should be able to devise a workable formula that suits your lifestyle. *As Ralph Waldo Emerson puts it, if you learn only methods, you will forever be tied to those methods, if you learn the principle behind those methods, you'll be free to devise your own method and become the master of your destiny and the author of your experience.* The echoes of those kind words are truly endless in my life, and we think you should be able to do the following with this book.

The pages of this book emphasize the following philosophy as you heal your liver:

- Decrease your viral load naturally with botanical antibiotics.
- Protect your liver and prevent further deterioration.
- Manage or prevent progress to liver cancer.
- Know about iron overload and hepatitis C.
- Optimize cellular levels of the most important antioxidant glutathione which makes liver detoxification possible.
- Stimulate regeneration of damaged liver cells.
- Reverse fibrosis and cure cirrhosis.
- Replace inflammation-damaged liver cells.
- Eat right and have your normal life expectancy.

- Know the herbs that will heal your liver.
- Use your mind and attitudes to heal your body.
- Containing the contagiousness of hepatitis B.
- Take care of the lymphatic system to increase immune function.

Chapter 1

Understanding Hepatitis and liver disease

What Is Hepatitis?

"Hepar" means liver in Greek and "itis" literally means inflammation. Hepatitis is inflammation of the liver precipitated by a wide variety of causes that includes viral attacks, inappropriate immune responses to chemical toxins (autoimmune hepatitis), environmental toxins, drugs, and alcohol (alcoholic hepatitis). An excerpt from *Healing Hepatitis Naturally* dates the first reported case of infectious liver disease, or jaundice, as far back as 751 A.D. Hyper-stimulation of the immune system in response to toxins and antigens is one of the major etiologies of inflammatory liver diseases, and taming liver inflammation is the most important prognostic tool in the management of hepatitis. *Liver inflammation is the driving force in the progression of chronic liver disease to liver cancer.*

"Great men are they who see that spiritual is stronger than any material force, that thoughts rule the world" Emerson

Contagious and Non-contagious Hepatitis

Hepatitis is either viral or non-viral. *Viral or contagious hepatitis* is caused by viruses with special affinities for human liver cells. Viral or contagious hepatitis is also referred to as *infectious hepatitis*. Non-viral hepatitis or non-contagious hepatitis is also referred to as *toxic hepatitis*. Contagious hepatitis exists in five forms, which are classified alphabetically: Hepatitis A, B, C, D, and E. Hepatitis A and E viruses cause acute hepatitis while the B, C and D viruses can lead to chronic infections. *Chronic hepatitis* is hepatitis infection lasting more than six months. Another type of hepatitis is called *fluminant hepatitis*; a severe and potentially-fatal form of acute hepatitis. Hepatitis viruses are opportunistic organisms that see liver inflammation as a chance to activate their mechanism. As we learn to take that opportunity away, we are steps ahead of infective hepatitis.

1

Treatment modalities that emphasize antiviral therapy over inflammation are like blaming the policemen for prisoners in the jail. The majority of inflammatory reactions in the body end with this medical suffix '-itis' and are not treated as infectious, e.g. iritis, pericarditis, colitis, uveaitis, dermatitis myocarditis, diverticulitis, rheumatoid arthritis, and tendinitis. It is not uncommon for individuals with liver inflammation to have latent inflammation going on in other parts of the body.

What Is A Virus?

A virus is a lifeless entity when independent, but alive under the right conditions. It is an opportunistic organism that is neither dead nor alive. They are thought to predate mankind. Viruses, unlike human cells and bacteria, are not independent living entities. They are unable to eat, grow, and reproduce. They lack the chemical equipment (enzymes) needed to carry out chemical reactions for life. Viruses only carry information needed to decode their genetic instructions. Therefore, a virus must have a host cell (e.g. a human, plant, or animal cell) in which to live and make more viruses. Once inside the body, viruses find a host cell to infect and regardless of the type of host cell, follow a basic cycle referred to as the *lytic cycle*:

The lytic cycle proceeds in the following steps:
1. A virus particle attaches to a host cell.
2. The particle releases its genetic material into the host cell.
3. The injected genetic material recruits the host cell's enzymes.
4. The enzymes make parts for more new virus particles.
5. The new particles assemble the parts into new viruses.
6. The new particles break free from the host cell.

Virology is the study of viruses, laboratory terminologies, and indices that identifies them. It identifies different stages of viral diseases and therapeutic interventions. Virology studies blood serum tests that show the presence of viral antigens, viral antibodies, and the phase of viral multiplication in the body. Any entity that has the ability to replicate uncontrollably under favorable condition is said to have viral characteristics. As an illustration, a stagnant stream is known to breed mosquitoes. The proliferation of mosquitoes will continue as long as stagnation exists. This type of situation is said to be *viral* and can be stopped not with insecticides but by changing the stream flow from stagnation to free flowing. The use of insecticides helps the mosquitoes develop an immunity which allows them to survive.

These characteristics are applicable to viruses, too, as they can develop resistant strains to elude antimicrobial agents that do not address the host's internal environment and immune system that makes viral contact infective.

What happens at first contact with a virus?

Nature has equipped the human body with many layers of protection against intruders or foreign bodies before they get in the blood stream and activate the immune system. These include the skin and the mucus membranes that line the mouth, ear, private parts, nostrils, lungs, the eyes, and the digestive tract. These membranes secrete antimicrobial agents that encounter microbes before they get into the blood stream. It is the breakdown in one or all of these defenses that lead to encounters with the immune system. These encounters are first picked up by the sensors nature puts in place to alarm the immune system, much like a home alarm system. When the immune system encounters an intruder, its sensors triggers the alarm system that activates chemical messengers to attack the intruders—a protective mechanism like the home-alarm monitoring company that calls the police to encounter the intruder.

These responses occur in two phases—cellular and oxidative.

Cellular responses

The cellular immune responses include the actions of chemical messengers called leukotrines and prostaglandins. Prostaglandins open the blood vessels for white blood cells to flow in and initiate the healing process. They also send pain messages to the brain by stimulating nerve endings. Leukotrines, like the Joint Chiefs of Staff in government, direct the activities of white blood cells at the site of infection. They orchestrate increased migration of white blood cells to the liver, where they filter intruders out of the blood while trying to restore homeostasis and normality. These migratory patterns are responsible for the warmth, heat, pain, and redness experienced during inflammation.

Under the direction of the leukotrines, kupffer cells, which are specialized liver cells, are the first to engage an invading virus. Kupffer cells serve as first responders or body guards in the liver. They are responsible for monitoring the liver for intruders such as the hepatitis virus. On contact with the hepatitis virus, they hold down the virus, break it into fragments, and signal the regulators of the immune system, the T-lymphocytes (Schmidt,

Smith and Sehnert, 1994). After T-lymphocytes are signaled for help, T-helper cells bind to the kupffer cells and lock onto viral antigens to form antigen-antibody complexes that interact with other subtypes of the T-cells to fight the invading virus. Other T-helper cells rush to the spleen and the lymph nodes for more T-helper cells to maintain the response while soliciting the immune system for other reinforcements.

The activated T-helper cells again stimulate the production and multiplication of other specialized types of T-cells called the T-killer cells, which attack the virus at the site of infection and kill infected host cells. The T-killer cells kill the host cells, infected by the hepatitis, by puncturing their membranes and letting the viral contents spill out, which hinders their usage for viral replication (Schmidt, Smith and Sehnert, 1994)

The activated T-helper cells also stimulate the production of B-cells that reside in the spleen which manufacture antibodies to destroy the virus. Meanwhile, under the actions of the leukotrines, interferons are produced which make the host cells, infected by the hepatitis virus, self destruct—nature's way of stopping the spread of infections.

In individuals whose immune or lymphatic systems are sluggish due to malnutrition or stress, the immune cells fail to launch the above defenses and the invading viruses use the host's genetic material to replicate themselves. In humans with healthy immune or lymphatic systems, the infection manifests only the acute phase and is localized to a part of the body, manifesting as stye, scar, or carbuncles after acute reactions to the invader. These responses deactivate the alarm and the war dwindles signifying recovery, Success!

As the war dwindles, the T-helper cells again send out the suppressor T-cells, a third type of the T-cells, to slow down or stop the activity of the B-cells and T-killer cells .They stop the attack of acute infections and encourage recovery. The memory cells are produced by the first exposure to infective agents. They stay in the blood stream for years and give lifelong immunity from subsequent infections and increase the response time to invasion by the same virus (Sehmidt, Smith and Sehnert, 1994).
Putting all the blame on the virus and combating hepatitis exclusively with antiviral actions is like making an accessory to a crime the prime suspect.

An aberrant virus, fungus, or bacteria in the body can only survive in an acidic environment (Baroody, 2002).

Currently, the FDA has not approved viral count as a diagnostic procedure; therefore it is only used for research purposes. The procedures for viral count are highly variable depending on the specific lab which performs the test. Different labs at different times almost always produce different results. Viral counts can change within a day or within a week. Efforts aimed at eliminating the virus at the cost of the patient's health are only short term. Along with these improvements is the deterioration of life. While synthetic alpha interferon and Reberton as anti-virals improve the lab markers and liver function tests, patients become sicker and weaker and their quality of life deteriorated (Quigcai Zhang, Zhang Clinic.)

⊠ *Flashback*

It is the failure and breakdown of this process and the immune – lymphatic system that made my Hepatitis virus attack infective and chronic.

Oxidative responses

The oxidative phase involves the movement or leakage of fluids, antibodies, and blood plasma from the blood vessels to the surrounding tissues which ultimately leads to swelling around the liver. The liver does not experience pain or discomfort. The swelling distends the surrounding tissues, compressing, irritating, and stimulating their nerve endings and causing the pain experienced during inflammation. Normally, this process is self-limiting and the individual may or may not experience minor symptoms of nausea, fever, vomiting, or mild scarring.

When the Infection Becomes Chronic

In chronic inflammatory liver disease, this process refuses to stop; the liver becomes a battle field like a California brush fire that spreads uncontrollably. In individuals with under-active immune systems, the alarm system fails to respond to the invader. Similarly, in cases of chronic inflammatory diseases, the alarm goes on and on initiating excessive responses that harm the host. Both of these scenarios constitute inappropriate responses of nature's response against pathogens and the host is caught in the middle. The damage caused by excessive response of the immune system further weakens the liver cells, making it possible for the invading virus to take advantage of this vulnerability and to replicate uncontrollably.

How is the liver damaged during viral infection?

During chronic inflammation, the liver often suffers from the friendly fires of these healing messengers that are directed at the pathogen (virus). The efforts directed by the white blood cells to counteract the virus end up on the liver. The responses from the immune system ultimately cause the damage associated with hepatitis, and the disruptions in the functions of the liver are elicited as the symptoms of hepatitis that includes elevated liver enzymes. This leaves localized scar tissues on the liver. If this continues unabated, scarring reduces the functional area and abilities of the liver. The scar is referred to as cirrhosis. What happens to fresh hamburger as it cooks on a grill is exactly how the cirrhotic process occurs. If the inflammatory fires are not abated, viruses thrive and liver cancer can ensue. The driving force in chronic hepatitis is the ability of the virus to break through the host immune defenses or weak cellular defenses and cause excessive immunological response that causes cirrhosis. Efforts directed solely at the microbes are purely misdirected for only one purpose-financial gains at the expense of thousands of lives lost in the war against infective diseases.

"Of one thing I am certain, the body is not a measure of healing; peace is the measure" George Melton

Where is the liver?

The liver is located in the right upper quadrant of the abdomen, just beneath the abdomen. It has two main lobes. Its base touches the right kidney, the stomach, and intestines. It weighs about three pounds. It has regenerative ability even if 75 percent of it is lost to illness. The adult liver weighs between 2 to 6 pounds and comprises one fifth of the total body weight. Beneath and attached to the liver is the gall bladder which is a small sac shaped like a pear. The bile ducts that spread out of the gallbladder like tree branches are referred to as bilary trees. They receive bile acids produced by the liver which are drained into the gall bladder.

The liver is the second largest organ in the body. (The skin is the largest organ.) It carries the greatest workload of all other organs. It is also about 95 percent water. Several times each day, our entire blood supply passes through the liver and about one pint of blood or 10 percent of the total blood volume is in the liver any time It is reddish brown in color and shaped like a cone.

The liver's blood supply The blood supply to the liver includes the hepatic artery that carries oxygenated blood. This oxygen-rich blood reaches the liver directly from the heart after passing through the lungs. The liver receives most of its blood from the portal vein. Blood from the portal vein does not reach the liver directly but passes first through the intestine, making it the first organ to have access to nutrients, drugs, and toxins absorbed from the stomach and the intestine. Nutrients and toxins from the digestive system get to the liver via this path. The portal vein is connected with the splenic vein, which drains the spleen. If blood flow is disrupted in the liver, there will be a back up in the spleen.

How does the liver utilize nutrients or toxins?

The liver cells are separated from each other by the sinusoids which under the microscope are seen to consist of rows of cells separated by spaces. The sinusoids are structured like a filter or sieve through which the blood is filtered. This space is highly vascularized with oxygenated blood from the hepatic artery and intestinal nutrients from the portal veins.

The hepatic artery and the portal vein enter the liver through a fissure at the base of the liver called the porta hepatic. From this point, the two blood vessels branch out to feed the right and left lobes of the liver. In the liver, the vessels keep dividing to become tiny branches, like a delta or a tree branch, to every part of the liver. These tiny branches drain into the sinusoids. The sinusoids allow compounds in the blood to have direct access with the hepatocytes, the cells of the liver where metabolism takes place. In the sinusoidal spaces, the kupffer cells, fat storing cells, and endothelial cells reside. This is where blood from the portal veins and hepatic artery mix.

The blood vessels that transverse the liver supply the liver with nutrients and toxins and the liver acts on these supplies by metabolizing, using, storing, and excreting them. It is in this space that nutrient exchange takes place.

Blood leaves the liver through the hepatic vein, which drains into the vena cava, which takes the blood to the heart.

What is the liver's job?

- All the food we eat, the air we breathe, the creams on our skin, the water we drink, and the drugs we take and everything we encounter in our environment passes through the liver.
- The liver manufactures about 14,000 chemicals, and uses about 60,000 systems and thousands of unknown synergistic activities. It converts the foods into biologically-active and usable forms for the body.
- The liver has the ability to set regeneration into process after chemical or physical insult within seven hours of insult.

- The liver employs amino acids as chemical building blocks to build several types of proteins that include blood clotting factors, biological materials, molecules, and tissues. This includes the synthesis and secretion of albumin that is necessary for maintaining proper fluid balance. Through the process of deamination and transamination the hepatocytes synthesize about 12 essential amino acids, remove ammonia from the body by the synthesis of urea, and convert the non-nitrogenous part of those molecules into glucose or lipids using the enzymes alanine and aspartate aminotransferases.
- The liver is essential for fat metabolism. The liver makes bile that breaks down fats through emulsification. The bile produced is stored in the gall bladder. During this process large fat molecules are metabolized into tiny water-soluble and absorbable droplets. (This is like the action of detergents that break down grease into tiny droplets which are rinsed off with water.) The bile is a vehicle for the elimination of toxic drugs and chemicals. The red blood cells protein hemoglobin is converted into bilirubin, which is greenish-yellow in color. In the liver, hepatocytes convert albumin-bound bilirubin in the blood into conjugated bilirubin and secretes it into the gall bladder through the bile duct into the liver for the metabolism of fats and fat soluble vitamins A, D, E, and K.
- Metabolism of alcohol, drugs, and detoxification of harmful substances takes place in the liver. The liver processes waste products and discharges them into the urine. It eliminates neutralized poisons into the bile and excretes it into the stool

as solid waste. It is responsible for converting essential thyroid hormone thyroxin into its more active form (T3). The liver is also responsible for removing ammonia, a toxic by-product of animal protein metabolism, breaking down hormones, including insulin which if it is not broken down fast enough continues to lower blood sugar levels, and neutralizes toxic chemicals from internal metabolic activities and from the environment.

- The liver is a nutrient warehouse for the storage of fats, sugars, vitamins, iron, and other nutrients, and sends them out as needed to body parts. It stores extra blood which is released in time of need. The liver is responsible for storing various nutrients, especially vitamins and iron, for release when needed. It helps stores fuel in the form of glycogen, which is released when the body needs it.

- The liver is responsible for homeostatic regulation of blood sugar levels, i.e. regulating the release of glycogen (stored sugar). When sugar is low, a healthy liver converts stored glycogen into glucose, releasing it into the blood stream to raise blood sugar levels. When sugar is high, a healthy liver will convert excess sugar into glycogen for storage.

- The liver maintains electrolyte and fluid balance in the body. The liver homeostatically maintains the level of sexual hormones.

- The liver is responsible for regulation of dietary proteins, synthesis of plasma proteins, synthesis of the inactive hormone angiotensinogen, and phagocytosis of damaged red blood cells, bacteria, etc. by the kupffer cells, absorption and breakdown of circulating hormones (insulin and epinephrine) and immunoglobulin. It also processes gas in the blood which is transferred to the lungs for removal.

What are Liver Enzymes?

•The liver has a lot of enzymes that serve as organic catalysts that boost many of the chemical reactions involving transformation and synthesis of nutrients that pass through the liver to usable and body-friendly states.

"Luck is a matter of preparation meeting opportunity" Oprah Winfrey

- The aminotransferases are enzymes responsible for the conversion of amino acids derived from food sources to proteins which are the building blocks of all the structures, organs, and tissues of the body.
- In liver diseases, when the liver cells are damaged or dying, these enzymes in the liver cells leak from the cell into the blood and are recorded as high in diagnostic tests.
- When these enzymes leak, the body is not able to manufacture proteins and a lot of bodily functions suffer. The test for these enzymes indicates the liver cells are dying and allowing the enzymes to leak into the blood stream
- These enzymes are the ALT (alanine aminotransferase) and AST (aspartate aminotransferase.) The former names for these enzymes are SGPT and SGOT.
- When the liver cells die and are replaced by fibrotic and scar tissues, they stop producing enzymes. ALT levels can also rise in response to medications in drug-induced hepatitis.
- In most cases, hepatocyte death correlates with increase of blood ALT and AST. Blood AST is elevated in other diseases like heart attacks and skeletal-muscle damage.

ALT (Alanine aminotransferase) is an enzyme produced by the liver cells. Its levels are raised when the liver cells are damaged or die as in cases of liver disease. As cells are damaged, ALT leaks into the blood stream .**ALT levels may correlate with the extent of cell death from inflammation.** These enzymes are also present in cells of other tissues in the body like the heart and skeletal muscles.

⊠ *Flashback*
My ALT (SGOT) had skyrocketed to 2,829 IU/L (international units per liter) from 1,471 IU/L in less than one month with normal ranges being less than 65 IU/L for adults. This was a clear indication that my liver cells were rapidly being destroyed by the invading viruses, and the functional liver enzymes used for its normal metabolic activities were leaking out of the liver cells into my blood and organs at an alarmingly high rate.

AST (Aspartate aminotransferase) is produced in the muscle and is also raised in cases of liver disease. High AST levels may also indicate ongoing cirrhosis, cancer, or alcoholic hepatitis.

⊠ *Flashback*

My AST was 644 IU/L when normal ranges are 15 – 37 IU/L. My ability to manufacture proteins from amino acids from food was hampered, and every major organ in my body was in a degenerative state. My total protein was 0.8 when normal range is 6.4 – 8.4.This indicated low levels of utilizable protein in my body despite being present in my system. It is like a fish being thirsty in the water. I had developed wasting muscle diseases .This caused the brittle nails, hair loss, and muscle wasting I suffered. The ongoing liver damage hampered the ability of my liver to manufacture blood-clotting factors. This decreased my ability to synthesize and secrete a variety of factors necessary for clotting. Consequently I bled profusely with minor scratches.

Alkaline phosphatese is a group of enzymes produced in the bile ducts, intestines, kidneys, placenta, and bones. Elevated alkaline phosphate indicates diseases of the bile ducts like primary biliary cirrhosis. It is found in cells of the bones, kidney, and intestine

⊠ *Flashback*

My alkaline phosphatese stood at the 203 when normal ranges are 50 – 136. This arises from marked obstruction in my bile ducts and cholestasis. My cirrhotic condition lead to enlargement of my spleen (splenomegaly) because the flow of blood through my liver was impeded. Consequently, my platelet count was consistently low because the platelets were being sequestered in the enlarged spleen. As a result on the ongoing cirrhosis, the blood vessels in my liver were seriously constricted and blood could not flow freely through my liver. Hence, there was a pressure build-up due to this backflow of fluids from my cirrhotic liver that resulted in portal hypertension. Over a five-month period, I had an average of 13 liters of fluids drawn from my abdomen at 15 different times through a process called parasynthesis. Before each round of parasynthesis, I would get intravenous administration of frozen plasma, platelets as clotting factors, and white blood cells since my blood counts were generally low. Parasnythesis is an invasive procedure and I ran a high risk of excessive bleeding and infections. I had several bouts of bacterial infections.

Gamma-glutamyltranspeptidase (GGPT) is present mainly in the parts of liver cells that produces bile and the bile ducts. High GGPT is also seen in individuals taking medications. High GGPT may mean blockage, inflammation, or damage to the bile ducts or disruption of bile flow in cholestasic liver diseases. Intrahepatic cholestasis indicates injury or blockage within the liver, like primary biliary cirrhosis or liver cancer, and extra-hepatic cholestasis refers to injury or blockage outside the liver. When the bile ducts are blocked or inflamed, GGTP overflows into the blood and is picked up as an elevated level in laboratory tests

High-alkaline phosphatase and GGTP with normal ALT and AST suggest bile duct disease or abnormal bile flow. Normal GGT level is 6 – 59 IU/L.

Bilirubin is a yellowish pigment that comes from the breakdown of hemoglobin, the oxygen-carrying molecules of red blood cells. It is transported out through the bile duct where it mixes with the wastes in the colon for onward excretion. Bilirubin is derived from the destruction of old red blood cells which are converted to bile through a conjugation process and stored in the gallbladder. From the gallbladder they are released to the intestine. When bilirubin concentrations in the blood are high, it is referred to as hyperbilirubinemia. If it is not cleared by the liver, it can produce jaundice in hepatitis. This means that more red blood cells are dying that are being replaced or the liver is injured and cannot convert bilirubin into bile. When concentrations of bilirubin are high, the kidney filters some of it. This turns the urine yellow or brown in color. The excess bilirubin turns the skin and whites of the eyes yellow, a condition called *jaundice*. The stools begin to look pale and white because bilirubin is lingering in the blood and tissues instead of being excreted into the stools. The stool loses its characteristic brown color.

☒ *Flashback*
My bilirubin level stood at 20 mg/dl for eight months when the normal range is 0.1 – 1.2 mg/dl. This was primarily due to significant liver damage and ongoing cirrhosis. While the red blood cells were being destroyed, my damaged liver could not convert them into bile through the conjugation process. Also, there was extreme blockage of my bile ducts due to the presence of gallstones in my gallbladder.

Albumin is the major protein that circulates in the blood stream. It is produced by the liver and secreted into the blood. Low albumin concentration indicates poor liver function. This signifies a wasting disease in which the body has proteins as food in the body but the diseased liver cannot utilize them as albumin. Albumin helps keep fluids in the blood vessels, hence preventing stomach, arm, and leg swelling. Unprocessed circulating amino acids in the body often leads to organ toxicity. This accounts for the swellings in arms, legs, stomach, and extremities seen in individuals with liver cirrhosis

☒ *Flashback*
Significant liver damage and cirrhosis brought my Albumin level to 2.8 for a period of six months when normal albumin levels are 3.4 – 5.0 g/dl .When albumin levels fall below 25 g/L, plasma diffuse from the veins and arteries into tissues. This clearly indicated that my liver cells could not perform one of their critical functions: utilization of proteins. As proteins are building blocks for every organ and tissues in the body, the inability to process proteins meant that I had progressed into the degenerative phase.

Prothrombin helps the blood to coagulate and clot. When the liver loses its ability to make clotting factors, blood levels of these factors are low and prothrombin time is prolonged. People with low prothrombin bruise and bleed easily like hemophiliacs. The prothrombin time indicates how long it takes the blood to clot. Normal prothrombin time is less than 15 seconds

Complete blood count (CBC). The CBC tests the degree of scarring of the liver and the presence of portal hypertension or back up of blood flow in the spleen. The spleen becomes enlarged. Platelets become trapped in the enlarged spleen, cannot enter the blood vessels, and the platelet count falls.

☒ *Flashback*
My cirrhotic condition caused me to be anemic and have low serum hemoglobin concentrations, which is an indication of the number of white blood cells. My laboratory tests consistently indicated low white blood cell count.

What are liver function tests?
Radiological imaging tests liver function and used to access the progression of liver disease. Each of these imaging tests has advantages and disadvantages relative to costs and amount of radiation associated with them.
- **The ultrasound or sonography** is a non-invasive and relatively inexpensive way to access the condition of the liver.

It uses high-frequency sound waves. Sound waves are sent to the liver and they bounce off liver tissues. The machine translates the sounds into visual images of the liver. It helps to isolate tumors, scars or cysts on the liver, patency of the bile ducts to rule out obstructions from stones, scars, or tumors. It provides clear images of the gall bladder. It is used for detecting gallstones. It also shows fluid build-up in the stomach. Since it does not involve radiation, it is safe for people who worry about radiation. However, sonograms cannot differentiate between a cancerous and non-cancerous tumor. If a sonogram appears normal, it does not totally rule out liver disease or liver cancer.

- **Computerized Axial Tomography (CAT scan or CT scan)** uses computerized tomography and low-level radiation to form a static image that is similar to an x-ray. It produces images based on x-rays taken from various angles. They offer more information than ultrasound as they generate more sharply-defined images that are not distorted by fluid or air. Clearer views give more consistent and actual assessments of liver problems like cirrhosis or tumors. The few possible side effects of CAT scans include allergic reactions to the intravenous contrast dyes administered before the test. They can cause acute kidney failure in individuals with liver problems, and can be used to measure the size of the liver. Like ultrasound, it can diagnose cirrhosis only if it is advanced and the liver is shrunken and nodular. It cannot be used to diagnose hepatitis or inflammatory diseases of the liver. The images produced show cross-sections of the liver architecture.
- **Magnetic resonance imaging (MRI)** makes use of magnetic fields and radio signals instead of radiation.
- **Endoscopy retrograde cholangiopancreatography (ERCP)** is used to see the bile ducts and gallbladder. An endoscope is inserted into the esophagus and passed into the small intestine under anesthesia. X-ray pictures are then taken.

☒ *Flashback*
Between 2002 and 2006, I had series of MRIs, CAT scans, ultrasounds, and countless x-rays which indicated I had an enlarged spleen, pre-cancerous cysts

all over my liver, cirrhotic morphology, blocked bile ducts, and less than 10 percent of usable liver function.

- **The liver biopsy** is an invasive procedure that involves the insertion of a needle directly into the liver and uses the needle to take a small sample of the liver tissue for histological evaluation. The procedure is done with local anesthesia. It is used to assess the presence or absence and extent of liver damage and to track the progression of the disease. Liver biopsy gives more accurate information at the cellular level about the extent of liver damage than a screening for liver cancer or other diseases that raises the level of liver enzymes to keep track of the health of the liver. It gives medical personnel an actual condition of the liver. It is used to determine the extent or stage of liver disease. Along with other tests like ultrasound or CAT scans, liver biopsy can be used to find the actual location of lesions, tumors, and cancers. The risks associated with biopsies includes bleeding, puncturing the lung, gall bladder, kidney or intestine, pain, infection, or inflammatory reaction to surgical instruments. Because an incision is made on the liver during biopsy, there is bleeding and scarring. Hence the risks and benefits should be carefully evaluated before doing the procedure. The results of the biopsy helps doctors indicate the *stage* of the disease.
- Stage I shows only inflammation of the liver with minimal scaring.
- Stage II indicate localized fibrosis; the scarring has developed and extended outside the portal tracts. These are the places that house the blood vessels in the liver. These are the areas where the inflammations starts.
- Stage III involves the spread of the fibrosis to neighboring tracts. The fibrosis is moderate to severe and connected by bridges of fibrous liver tissues.
- Stage IV indicate the progression of the fibrosis to cirrhosis, and liver function is compromised.

After a biopsy test had been done and the stage of hepatitis infection obtained, other blood tests that measure the white blood cells, hemotocrit, platelets, prothrombin, complete blood count, bilirubin, albumin, clotting factors, enzyme levels (ALT, SGOT, Alkaline Phosphate), and hormonal levels are aggregated to assess the true condition of the liver.. The totality of the above tests should tell the state of the liver, how much inflammation is going on, and how much liver damage has occurred. This will guide attending personnel in selecting a line of therapy.

Chapter 2

What are the types of liver diseases?

Contagious Hepatitis

Bacteriologists are unanimous in declaring that the various disease germs are found not only in diseased bodies but also in the bodies of seemingly health persons. All disease germs known to medical science are found in humans as young as two month olds. (Henry Lindlahr MD)

- In the 1940s, two routes of infectious hepatitis were established: food-borne and blood-borne
- Hepatitis A is food borne hepatitis, i.e. caused by a food-borne virus
- Hepatitis B, C, and D are classified as blood-borne i.e. transmitted via a blood-borne virus
- Hepatitis B and C are classified as serum hepatitis since they are transmitted through infected blood or blood products

Hepatitis A Virus (HAV)

According to the Center for Disease Control, Hepatitis A, or HAV, accounts for 25 percent of all viral hepatitis in the United States. Approximately 140,000 *"If a window of opportunity appears, don't pull down the shade" Tom Peters* people are infected annually with HAV in the United States. About 30 percent of all people in the United States have been infected with HAV. The incubation period—the time between initial exposure and manifestation of symptoms—is about 30 days. Contamination comes from infected food, water polluted with infected fecal matter, contaminated foods, vegetables, and sea foods, like shell fish, which are often caught in contaminated water. Infection can also come through anal sex, oral sex, kissing, recreational IV drug use, and eating raw foods. HAV manifests only acute symptoms that include fatigue, jaundice, fever, nausea, abdominal pain, light stool, and dark urine. People with chronic infective hepatitis can have HAV. Infected children do not manifest any apparent liver disease. Severe liver infection can be life-threatening in adults. HAV is diagnosed with the presence of antibodies to the virus in blood by obtaining a specific blood test known as hepatitis A serology. People with HAV may have elevated liver enzymes and bilirubin. Inactivated hepatitis A vaccine is often used in management of HAV. This vaccine is recommended for those traveling to high-risk areas and for people with chronic hepatitis B, C or HIV/AIDS. The vaccination prevents HAV infection in adults and children older than two years. An initial dose followed by a booster dose six months later offers protection for 10 – 20 years. The CDC recommends vaccination for people traveling to developing countries like Africa, Asia (except Japan), Europe, the Middle East, central and South America, and the Caribbean. Once an individual recovers from HAV, there is lifetime immunity. The best prevention against HAV is personal hygiene. There is a fatality rate of about 45 percent among people who have Hepatitis C or who are HIV positive.

Hepatitis B Virus (HBV)
The hepatitis B virus (HBV) is a single molecule of DNA or RNA in a protein coat. Like other viruses, it is a microscopic organism that cannot perform any living functions on it's own until it infects a host liver cell. And it has to get pass the immune system to infect a liver cell.

"If you bring forth what is inside you, what you bring forth will save you" – The Gospel According to Thomas

Who Discovered HBV?
During the Second World War, yellow fever vaccines given to army recruits were mistakenly contaminated with viruses that elicited jaundice. Further investigations found the viruses to be hepatitis. The HBV was discovered by Dr Baruch Blumberg, a Nobel Prize winner in 1965, while studying the genetic correlation to diseases and how antibodies react to antigens. Dr. Blumberg did his test by collecting blood samples from different indigenous tribes worldwide. He observed that antibodies from some people in the Australian aborigine reacted against an antigen. In 1966, he corroborated his findings with virologist Alfred Prince of the New York Blood Center who was doing some work on transfusion. Prince believed that the Australian antigen Blumberg had discovered was related to the HBV.

In 1967, the Australian antigen was confirmed to be the HBV. It was initially called the AU or Australian antigen. In 1986, the HBV was first observed under an electron microscope and the first samples were grown in test tubes. (Green, 2002). It was determined that the Australian antigen was a surface antigen for the Hepatitis B virus (HBsAg). This surface antigen is a protein synthesized by the virus DNA genetic material and is an important element in the virus coat. In1972, the FDA mandated all blood banks to screen blood received for the HBV virus. In 1973, the American Association of Blood Banks followed the FDA mandate and adopted the test. Since 1975, more sensitive tests have been introduced; however, individuals who received blood transfusions before 1975 may have come into contact with the HBV and should be tested for it.

How Widespread is HBV Virus in the USA?
- The Centers for Disease Control estimate that the HBV virus affects more than one million people in the United States, with 200,000 new cases added annually. However, most individuals fight off the infection and gain lifelong immunity.
- One in 20 Americans will be infected with Hepatitis B at some point in their lives. The majority will elicit no symptoms or will manifest only mild flu-like symptoms. While most people recover, a little over 1 million people remain chronically infected with HBV in the United States. This translates to one in every 200 Americans.
- Between 4,000 to 5,000 people die each year in the United States from complications of HBV virus.
- The American Liver Foundation indicates that well over 40 percent of people infected with HBV virus are unaware of it and do not show noticeable symptoms. While doctors routinely test for the HIV virus, the opposite is the case for HBV. For every individual that is HIV positive, there are ten HBV-positive people.

How Global is the HBV Epidemic?
- HBV is endemic in places like New Zealand, Sub Saharan Africa, Australia, South America, and the Middle East.

- HBV is the number one cause of liver disease worldwide. About 70 percent of the world's populations have had contact with HBV at some point in their life.
- There are about 2 billion people infected with HBV worldwide and 350 million people suffering from chronic HBV infections or about 5 percent of the world's population. HBV is the ninth leading cause of death worldwide.
- Between 500,000 to 1.2 million people die annually from chronic HBV and its complications. In Asia and most African countries, HBV infection is common and acquired prenatally or in childhood.

The World Health Organization states the following:
- HBV accounts for about 83 percent of all instances of liver cancer in the world.
- Two thirds of the world population has been infected with HBV at some time in their lives.
- Over one million people die each year from HBV-related complications.
- About 550,000 people worldwide die each year from liver cancer.
- One out of every four people with chronic hepatitis B will die from cancer or liver cirrhosis.

How is Hepatitis B Transmitted?
HBV is transmitted through body fluids, including blood, semen, vaginal secretions, saliva, and any break in the skin and mucous membranes.

HBV modes of transmission include the following:
- Blood transfusions or contaminated blood products
- Unprotected homosexual or heterosexual sex. (HBV is 100 times more contagious that HIV. The risk of contracting HBV is 30 times greater via a needle stick than Hepatitis C virus.
- Illicit drug use, e.g. snorting cocaine with shared straws and/ or needles.)
- Getting Tattoos with unsterilized needles
- Having a hair cut or shaving with unsterilized instruments
- Having a manicure or pedicure with unsterilized instruments

- Body piercing with unsterilized instruments
- Clinical accidents
- Infected mother-to-newborn–baby transmission via breast milk and in the birth canal
- Health care workers exposed to blood
- Organ transplantation
- Having dental work done with improperly sterilized equipments
- Sharing tooth brush, razors, or beauty-care utensils with infected persons
- Sharing pre-chewed foods
- Dialysis patients
- Since the Hepatitis B virus can stay alive for up to 10 days, even on a dry surface, it is important not to torch any blood, even if it is dry. All blood should be cleaned with a solution of one part household bleach to ten parts of water.

You cannot get hepatitis B from the following routes:
- air
- hugging
- sneezing
- coughing
- toilet seats
- doorknobs

You are at risk of contracting Hepatitis B if any of the following are true:
- you have unprotected sex with someone infected with the virus
- you have multiple sex partners
- You engage in homosexual sex, e.g. anal sex, oral sex, etc.
- you live with someone with chronic hepatitis B
- you have a job that involves contact with blood products
- you use illegal drugs
- You travel to high risk areas without vaccination.

What Does HBV Look Like?
Hepatitis B is a DNA virus and a member of the hepadnaviridae family of viruses that have affinity for liver cells. The infectious ("Dane") particle is comprised of an inner core protein plus an outer surface protein coat.

The outer shell is composed of several proteins called HBs, or surface proteins. The outer surface coat surrounds an inner protein shell composed of HBc, core proteins. The inner shell is called the core particle or capsid. The core particle surrounds the viral DNA and the enzyme DNA polymerase. The entire virion is known as a Dane particle. The HBV genome encodes a DNA polymerase that also acts as a reverse transcriptase. After the viron enters the liver cells, it is uncoated and its genome is delivered into its nucleus where it releases its contents of DNA and DNA polymerase into the liver cell nucleus. There the viral genome is converted into covalently closed circular DNA (cccDNA), a mitochromosome that serves as the viral transcription template .RNA serves as a pre-genomic template for reverse transcription to negative-strand DNA, which in turn becomes the template for transcription of positive-strand DNA. The mRNA transcribes viral proteins as well as pre-genomic RNA that is reverse transcribed into the HBV DNA of new virons. Without the reverse transcriptase, new virons cannot be produced and replication ceases.

The significance of this replicative strategy led to the development of drugs called nucleoside analogues that can block viral multiplication. Like most viruses, the HBV is a microscopic single molecule of DNA or RNA wrapped in a protein coat. It is an invisible parasite that cannot perform any living functions on its own until it infects a host cell. It has to get pass the immune system to infect a liver cell.

What Happens When One Comes In Contact With HBV?
When the "lifeless" hepatitis B virus get past the immune system to incorporate itself into the host cell and uses the DNA materials of the liver cells to replicate itself, it "comes alive." In the process the host cells become infected. Like an intruder using your home as it's staging ground, once the virus attacks a host cell, it takes over the machinery the cell and uses it to replicate itself. In the case of liver cells, the virus causes the liver cell's DNA or RNA to reproduce itself instead of the liver cells. A parasitic relationship now exists that benefits the HBV. The virus uses the liver's DNA as a template to replicate itself. The liver cells making the virus are referred to as "host infected cells." Thousands and millions of copies of the virus cells burst from the host liver cell, killing the liver cells in the process. Each new virus contaminates another host cell to make more copies. This explains how the virus moves around the liver.

How Does the HBV Virus Reproduce?
When the virus enters the body of a new host its initial response, if it gets past the immune system, is to infect a liver cell.

Knowing Laboratory Terminology
- *Seroconversion*, as the name implies, is the conversion of the antigens and/or antibodies from one form to another in blood serum. The forms can be positive or negative. This manifestation is used to assess the progression of the disease or its response to remedies. It may involve losing an antibody or gaining an antigen. When one loses antigens and gains antibodies in the serum, it indicates a favorable prognosis. In serological testing, various relationships between the antibodies and the antigens are used as prognostic tools to follow the progression of hepatitis and treatment response. This is called a lab-based approach.

  Monitoring lab markers for the antibodies and antigens are very crucial to accessing the body's response to the inflammation, the Hepatitis virus and it's treatment"

  John Imevbore

- *Antigens (Ag)* are protein signals or indicators on the surface of intruding virus cells that the host's immune system recognizes. They elicit immunological responses from the host they are invading since the immune system identifies them as foreign.
- *Antibodies (Ab)* are proteins produced by the white blood cells to fight antigens. (*Note*: Antigens are our foes, and antibodies are our friend.)
- The *"e" antigen* is a peptide discovered in 1973 that assists the HBV to higher levels of contagiousness. It is not a favorable presence. It has a protein coat that protects the infected liver cells from the immune system so the liver cells can house the HBV for a longer period of time. Its presence means HBV is actively multiplying. Remedies that can help the host to loose the "e" antigen are most beneficial. Loosing the "e" antigen is a favorable prognosis. The "e" antigen and its antibody, written as HBeAg and HBeAb, are antigens and antibodies seen in chronic and acute phases of hepatitis B infections.

- The *HBsAg surface antigen* to the hepatitis B virus indicates the liver is infected with HBV and the liver is producing the antigen. It also indicates that the host is contagious. These surface antigens and antibodies are the first indicators of initial infection, but their presence does not tell whether the infection is acute or chronic.

- *Core antigen and antibody*, HBcAg and HBcAb, are also known to as IgM anti HBc and IgG anti –HBc. They are usually not part of routine testing in hospitals and labs. The core proteins are part of the virus particle and constitute part of the viral coat that covers its nuclear material. When the virus establishes itself in the liver cells, this core protein is produced and the immune system responds to its presence by producing core antibodies. The presence of antibodies to core antigens in the blood is used to differentiate an acute from a chronic infection. The *core antigen* is the part of the virus that stimulates immunological response from the host liver cells. (*Note*: The "e" antigens and core antigens are produced by the virus during viral replications. Their presence indicates there is replication or multiplication of the virus.)

- *DNA polymerase* is an enzyme that helps release the hepatitis B DNA needed for the multiplication of hepatitis B virus. They are part of the virus's DNA and are released during active infection and replication of the virus. It can be used to monitor response to antiviral therapy.

What Are Immunoglobulins?

During encounters between the host immune system and the invading virus, the host antibodies lock on to the virus-surface antigens to form antigen – antibody complexes. This "tying up" of the virus antigens enable the immune system to take its time to organize the response needed to dispose the virus. These antibodies that lock on to the antigens are called immunoglobulins or Ig for short. In HBV infections, the IgG and IgM indicate the presence of antibodies that indicate ongoing or previous infections. People with IgG and surface antibodies for the HBV indicate the infection is resolved in them. Similarly individuals with IgG with no surface antibodies for the HBV have chronic HBV and are considered contagious. IgM are indicators of acute infections.

What Is Fluminant Hepatitis B?

Fluminant hepatitis B is a rare type of hepatitis B that manifests as sudden liver failure, bleeding propensity, jaundice, and encephalopathy coma. It is a progressive degenerative type of hepatitis B and fatal in about 85 percent of cases. It requires immediate liver transplant. Co-infection with other types of hepatitis is a risk factor for fluminant hepatitis B (Palmer, 2004).

Will I Overcome Hepatitis B Infection?

- About 90 percent of adults get rid of the virus, while about 10 percent will become chronic carriers. Unlike the hepatitis C virus, the hepatitis B virus does not mutate rapidly so antivirals and the immune system can launch a coordinated war against the virus.
- About 40 percent of young children will get rid of the virus and about 60 percent will end up as chronic carriers. About 90 percent of infants will become chronic carriers and about 10 percent of infants will be able to get rid of the virus

Phases of HBV

The immune system may accommodate the HBV virus in the host's blood. This occurs mostly in congenital cases or in teenagers because the immune system is developing or maturing and does not know what to do with the virus. This immune-tolerance phase may last into the adult years. It is followed by the immune clearance phase. This stage is characterized by the maturing immune system awakening and making an effort to clear the virus if it can. Favorable seroconversions can occur, but if not, the illness progresses to more chronic manifestations.

What Happens During Acute HBV Infection?

The disruption of the host's liver cells functions leads to acute symptoms of nausea, vomiting, fever, pain in the liver area, fatigue, dark urine, light stool, and jaundice. Infected cells leak their contents, which are read in laboratory tests as elevated liver enzymes. The HBV infection usually takes an average of two to eight weeks before the liver enzymes ALT and AST are elevated. The HBV virus infection is acute as long as the host immune system clears the virus and develops antibodies against it. Viral and immune indicators are detectable in the blood and the antibody – antigen markers are used to characterize the patterns of HBV infection.

The hepatitis B virus's surface antigens HBsAg, the surface protein of the HBV, also known as anti-HBs, are found in sweat, blood, saliva, semen, vaginal fluids, breast milk, tears, and nasal secretions. Appearance in the blood occurs from one to six weeks after initial infection and even before symptoms manifests. They are the first detectable viral marker of the illness. A positive test for the presence of these surface antigens is the standard test for an ongoing infection. Their presence indicates that there is HBV in the body of the individual. The Hepatitis B viral infection has an incubation period of 45 – 160 days. The average incubation period is 100 days

The HBsAg is followed by the HBeAg and HBV DNA. When the core of HBV disintegrates in the blood serum, the antigen is formed and detected by lab tests. This is found in the acute stage and resolves when the acute infection is over. If these antigens appear in the blood for more than six month, it indicates chronic infection. The titers are usually high during the incubation period but gradually level off. The hepatitis B viral DNA and hepatitis "e" antigen levels may continue to drop. During active infections, these immune-globulins (Ig) fuse with the hepatitis B surface antibody (HBsAb) to neutralize HBV infection. The presence of immunoglobulins in the blood and the time intervals between the disappearance of hepatitis B surface antigen (HBsAg) and the appearance of the antibodies-Anti-HBs is the standard marker for an acute infection. This time interval is referred to as the window period.

The most sensitive indicator of HBV replication is HBeAg. Laboratory tests that indicate the presence of HBsAg and IgM core antibody or core antibody alone during the window period are indicators of an acute infection. The loss of HBsAg and the presence of HBsAb imply recovery from the acute illness and development of immunity.

Immunity against HBV confers protection from hepatitis D but not hepatitis A and C. During the stages of rapid replication of the HBV virus, short forms of hepatitis B core antigen (HBeAg) are also found in the blood. HBV "e" antigen is derived from the core or a portion of the core of the HBV. The hepatitis B surface antibodies (HBsAb) to the virus are produced by the immune-globulins and secreted by the body's B lymphocytes in response to the presence of HBeAb, the Hepatitis antigen.

It appears after the test for HBeAg turns negative, signifying resolution of infection. And the presence of antibodies to hepatitis "e" (HBeAb) indicates a favorable prognosis.

⊠ *Flashback*
By August 2003, my Hepatitis B viral load was greater than 200 million copies per mL of blood when normal ranges were supposed to be less than 2,000 copies per mL of blood. I was highly contagious. This indicates that my viral load was too high to count by conventional diagnostic indices which disqualified me as a candidate for transplantation. My progression from acute to chronic phase of hepatitis B viral infection is thought to be primarily due to lack of vigorous T and B cells responses from the immune system.

When Does HBV Infection Becomes Chronic?
- The presence of HBsAg in the blood for more than six months indicates a chronic infection.
- The presence of IgG core antibodies indicates a chronic infection.
- Chronic HBV carriers are divided into two distinguishable states of HBV infection. The presence or absence of hepatitis B "e" Antigen (HbeAg) in the blood.
- In most cases of chronic infection, HBeAg is not detectable in the blood, i.e. the virus switches from a high-replicative detectable state to a low-replicative undetectable state.

When Is HBV Contagious?
When HBsAg, the hepatitis B surface antigen in the blood, is positive, HBV is contagious. When anti-HBc, the antibody to hepatitis B core antigen, is positive in the blood, infection is recent or occurred earlier. In other cases, if HBsAg is positive but the "e" antigen and Hepatitis B DNA is negative, no replication is going on but the individual is still contagious. If the "e" antigen and HB DNA are negative, contagiousness is reduced. High viral loads and a positive antigen "e" result indicate a serious contagious phase. When tests indicate the presence of the "e" antigen with HBV actively in the blood stream, the individual is still contagious. If tests indicate antigen "e" negative and *undetectable* HBV in the blood, the individual is not contagious, but could be infectious to some degree due to the possibility of seroconversion.

27

In summary:
- Individuals with HBsAg and HBeAg are highly contagious. They are undergoing active viral replication and are considered highly infective.
- Individuals are HBeAg negative and HBeAb are less contagious.
- Individuals with HBeAg negative, HB DNA negative, and HBeAb positive are not contagious.
- Inactive chronic carriers have HBeAb i.e. antibodies to the "e" antigens in their blood. Most people who are chronically infected are infected as infants because the immune systems of infants do not produce enough antibodies to eradicate the virus.

Who Are Healthy HBV Carriers?
- About 10 percent of HBV patients could not eradicate the virus after six months of infection, and about 80 percent of congenital HBV sufferers are chronic carriers.
- Inactive healthy carriers are persons infected with HBV but with no clinical evidence of infection. They have detectable hepatitis B surface antigens (HBsAg) in their blood but no signs or symptoms of liver disease.
- They show no signs of viral replication.
- They have laboratory evidence of HBV infection but no physical manifestation of the disease. *"About 75% of chronic carriers will have no evidence of inflammation on liver biopsy. They are referred to as true carriers. About 25% of chronic carriers show evidence of liver inflammation on liver biopsy. They are not true carriers. They have chronic hepatitis despite normal laboratory tests and no visible symptoms. They may exhibit liver cirrhosis on liver biopsy. They may develop clinically apparent hepatitis later in life."* (Worman, 1999).

Since one in four chronic carriers will die from complications of liver cirrhosis or liver cancer, early detection is crucial to prevent these complications.

WHO is a Silent Carrier?
Hepatitis B virus is referred to as "silent infection" because chronically-infected people can be infected for a long time and not be aware of it and

do not display any apparent symptoms of the disease. Such people often show up in the doctor's office with end-stage liver disease. Silent carriers have laboratory markers that test HBsAg positive with near normal liver enzymes, with low or no viral loads, and no symptoms of the disease.

The presence of HBeAg in the blood indicates an ongoing inflammation, high infective state, and higher chances of progression to cirrhosis and cancer if the inflammation becomes uncontrollably chronic. Since 1987, the rate of acute HBV infection has dropped because of the introduction of immunization of neonates, vaccinations of occupationally-exposed persons, refinements in the blood-donor screening, the use of virus-inactivated blood products for patients with bleeding disorders, and changes in lifestyles in high risk groups (Steeff, 1997).

How Do I Know If I Have Recovered from HBV Infection?

Individuals who get rid of the HBV virus lose the HbsAg indicator. Lab results show the presence of hepatitis B surface antibodies (HBsAb or anti-HBs.) They develop lifelong immunity. The presence of anti-HBsAb and anti-HBcAb (IgG) indicate recovery and immunity in a previously-infected person or have acquired immunity by receiving antibodies from their mother as infants. Vaccinations can cause the HBsAb, the Hepatitis B surface antibody marker, to be positive which can exist in the body for a long period of time.

Can I be Cured of Chronic Hepatitis b infection?

From a conventional point of view, cure is the reduction of the viral load to undetectable levels with anti-virals and/or interferon therapy. Like all other viruses that exist in the body, it is impossible to completely eliminate them from the organs. Tests that indicate undetectable levels in the blood and body fluids cannot test for their presence in the body tissues. In most instances, they go into a low-replicative phase and are not picked up by the most sensitive lab tests. This is why HBV is sometimes called an occult illness.

From a holistic point of view, involvement with religion, lifestyles changes in nutrition, botanical supplements, and stress reduction that help improve the quality of life, strengthen the terrains of the human body against viral onslaught, and arrest inflammation with active involvement of the host that ultimately leads to healing. Conventional and/or alternative protocols can sometimes lead to seroconverion in chronic hepatitis-B individuals. In those situations, individuals will need to monitor their blood work periodically as indicated by their physician for the rest of their lives to ensure that they remain non- contagious. Developing antibodies (HBsAb) to the hepatitis B virus, either through vaccination or through warding off acute infection, confers lifelong immunity for the hepatitis B viral infection. The hepatitis B viruses can remain undetectable with the use of hepatic herbs.

Doctors Health advisory: Individuals with HBV need to check for the presence of HIV, HCV, and HDV as co-infections. Individuals who continue to actively replicate the HBV virus with high levels of HBV DNA and HBeAg have progressive liver diseases with a high probability of progressing to cirrhosis, end-stage liver diseases, and hepatocellular carcinoma. Loss of the HBeAg does not mean permanent resolution of Hepatitis B infection.

What are the Conventional Treatments for Chronic Hepatitis B?
The use of synthetic drugs kills our incentives to find the root cause of our diminished immunity that make hepatitis B infective. In addition, such usage adds to the body's toxic loads. While antiviral agents treat the problem and not the person, botanical supplements treat both the person and the problem, the virus. Using antiviral therapies is like spraying your pantry for ants and leaving the open sugar jar on the shelf. Other ants will always come back for the sugar. Antibiotics are not used against viral infections because viruses like the HBV live inside their host's cell .For antibiotics to get to the virus they have to first destroy the liver cells, which is often too much collateral damage.

Drugs used in the management of hepatitis B with drugs falls into two categories:
- *Immune modulators, namely recombinant interferon alfa-2b*: The synthetic interferon alfa-2b was approved in the United States in 1992 as a therapy for chronic HBV. Its mode of action is to mimic natural interferons. Exogenous alpha interferon fails to resolve chronic HBV in many patients, and the therapy is often fraught with a variety of adverse reactions like other synthetic drugs, which includes low neutrophil and platelet

counts. The platelet count the body needs to fight infections is lowered by synthetic alpha interferon. In the short term, it is tolerated in less than 30 percent of hepatitis B patients. The majority of these patients relapse with discontinuation of interferon. To ameliorate adverse reactions from interferons, physicians generally recommend acetaminophen (Tylenol™). Liver damage from excessive use of acetaminophen is responsible for a majority of liver transplants in the United States. Exogenous interferon aggravates diabetes and thyroid disorders. It interferes with the nervous system, causing tingling in the hands, feet, arms, and legs. It causes depression, anxiety, irritability, confusion, nervousness, impaired concentration, insomnia, and suicidal ideation. Other more-frequent side effects include back pain, dry mouth, diarrhea, and inflammation at injection sites.

- **Inhibitors of HBV replication** (Lamivudine/Epivir and Adefovoif Dipivoxil/Hepsera.) These drugs prevent viral multiplication in the liver cells. They are aimed at preventing viral replication and prevention of end-stage liver disease. The markers of successful treatment with these drugs are HBeAg seroconversion, reduced or undetectable HBV DNA, and lack of disease progression.

How do synthetic antivirals Work?
When the HBV enters the host cell and takes control of the DNA it is converted to covalently-closed circular DNA. This serves as a template for a series of reverse transcriptions. From a clinical point of view, this reverse transcription strategy is what currently-available antiviral drugs disrupt. While they disrupt viral replication in infected liver cells, they also indiscriminately disrupt the enzymes systems of healthy liver cells, causing serious adverse reactions. The severity, types, and number of these adverse reactions are unpredictable. We want you to know that all hepatitis antiviral drugs cause hepatitis.

Lamivudine (Epivir,) also known as 3TC, is a nucleoside analog introduced in 1999. It inhibits the reverse transcriptase DNA polymerase of the HBV virus. The activity of this enzyme is essential for the replication of the virus. It is also used for the treatment of HIV infection. The HIV has a DNA polymerase also called reverse transcriptase that is inhibited by Lamivudine.

It is administered orally while interferon is administered by injection. Among all the FDA approved anti-viral drugs, Epivir is the best tolerated. Known side effects include loss of appetite, neuropathy, depression, skin rash, itching, bone aches, coughing, nervousness, diarrhea, fatigue, and headaches. It can cause abnormally high levels of acid in the blood, causing lactic acidosis, severe hepatomegally, and hepatitis. Abnormal laboratory test results due to Epivir include low red blood cells count, neutropenia (low white blood cell count), low platelet count, increased liver enzymes (ALT), and swollen lymph glands. Like all antiviral therapies, the HBV virus does mutate and become resistant to Epivir. Hence, there are at least 20 new anti-virals released annually in the United States because the HBV virus always mutate to new species to elude currently available anti-virals. It is worth knowing that viruses do not mutate against all available botanical antiviral and antibiotic herbs, many of which have been in existence as long as life itself. They do not have generics and were never modified. They are not marketed by pharmaceutical companies because they are available from natural sources.

Adefovir Dipivoxil (Hepsera) can suppress HBV strains that developed resistance to Epivir. The FDA approved it in 2002. Hepsera can cause worse or very serious hepatitis in some people when they stop taking it. It can also cause liver enlargement and damage. The warning signs include yellowing of the skin or eyes, dark urine, light colored stool, nausea, lower stomach pain, and loss of appetite for several days. Hepsera also causes kidney damage and lactic acidosis in some individuals. Lactic acidosis is a medical emergency. It's warning signs includes weakness, tiredness, unusual muscle pain, difficulty breathing, stomach pain, nausea, vomiting, cold feelings in the arms and legs, dizziness, or irregular heartbeat. In individuals with untreated HIV, Hepsera may increase the chances that the HIV infection cannot be helped with the usual HIV medicines. When Hepsera is discontinued, hepatitis can come back with more vigorous symptoms. Cummings and Ullman (2004) believes that if drugs are used to suppress conditions, when the drug effects wears off, the suppression often forces the body to create deeper symptoms to handle the underlying imbalance

The HBV is never completely eradicated from the body. It goes to a low-replicative phase, which is undetectable by blood tests. It can stay undetectable with strong immunity and the absence of stressors.

⊠ *Flashback*

My antiviral drug was switched from Epivir, Hepsera, and Viread to Baraclude. These drugs exacted such a tremendous toll on my liver and well being that I had to be weaned off of them for a few months. The liver pain, exacerbation of my liver enzymes, impaired kidney function, lactic acidosis, muscle cramps, and nausea associated with their use were managed with a low-salt diet and diuretics like Spironlactone (Aldactone) and Furosemide (Lasix.) I eventually discontinued their use against my doctor's advice in lieu of botanical antibiotic and liver-rescue herbs which reduced my viral loads safely. I went through seroconversion and my viral loads became undetectable.

What are the Facts about the Hepatitis B Vaccine?

The rational behind vaccination is the assumption that when a genetically-engineered, weakened living or dead virus is injected into the body, it will trick the body into producing antibodies to the disease. This is what happens when the body contracts the illness naturally. The duration of the immunity in the development of mutant strains and the adverse reactions from taking multiple injections are a two of the unknown variables.

In the development of HBV vaccine, it is important to note that the availability of successful immunoprophylaxis will not be useful to individuals who have developed chronic infections.

After discovering the HBV, Dr Blumberg and his colleague Irvin Millman, invented the first HBV vaccine (Green, 2002). The first vaccine was the inactivated or denatured HBV, which used heat to denature the HBV antigen. This vaccine elicited unwanted immunological responses. In 1973, plasma-derived vaccines were developed by collecting antibodies from individuals who overcame the HBV viral infection. Initially, the HBV vaccine was derived from the blood products of homosexual men who had hepatitis. These serum-based vaccines were later (1990) replaced with genetically-engineered or recombinant-DNA versions that are grown on yeast cells. The vaccines are given in three shots over a 6 – 12 month period, and they are thought to confer immunity for between 6 and 12 years. The majority of individuals who get the first shots are protected against the HBV virus, but full protection is only achieved after getting the complete series of shots.

Who needs to be vaccinated?

- Pregnant women
- All newborns needs to be vaccinated immediately after birth to deter complications associated with infections later in life.
- All individuals living with chronically-infected individuals
- All children and adolescents should be vaccinated against the HBV virus.
- Babies born to infected mothers are at higher risk of contracting hepatitis B virus. They should be given the hepatitis B immune-globulin and the hepatitis B vaccine within 12 hours after delivery to protect the new born baby from being infected. This should be followed by two additional doses at six and twelve months of age
- Any one with chronic liver disease
- Health care workers who handle blood and blood products.
- Individuals with hepatitis C and/or HIV infections.
- People undergoing hemodyalysis, IV drug users, family members and co- workers of infected persons, sexual partners of infected persons, nurses, doctors, laboratory workers, people who engage in risky sexual behaviors, people with multiple sex partners, and people who plan to travel to high risk areas. It is important for people who work regularly with infected persons to check their antibody levels and make sure it is above 10 units per mL. If antibody levels fall below this level, they need to get booster shots.
- Individuals who are unvaccinated and exposed to the HBV virus through blood or body fluids should get the intramuscular injection of hepatitis B immunoglobulin (HBIG) within 14 days of exposure followed immediately by the hepatitis B vaccine.

What are likely Adverse Reactions of HBV vaccines?

The body sees genetically-engineered products as foreign. In the process, the body elicits auto immune responses that can lead to wide varieties of auto-immune diseases. This is what accounts for the majority of the adverse reactions associated with vaccination. Side effects suffered by children vaccinated with the HBV vaccine include lethargy, malaise, asthma, diarrhea, arthritis, faintness, pallor, loss of consciousness, and drop in blood pressure. Between 1990 and 1994 about 12,000 adverse events linked to the HBV vaccine were reported in the United States. Anywhere from 30 – 50 percent of those vaccinated with the HBV vaccine will need booster shots every five years for the rest of their lives. The major problem with vaccination is eradication of one strain of a virus encourage other forms to proliferate new diseases from vaccines. (Mctaggart, 1996). Improved sanitation, education, stress reduction, hygiene, better nutrition, housing, and quarantine procedures also played noble roles in the eradication of communicable diseases

☒ *Flashback*
I was not eligible for the hepatitis B vaccine because I had already been infected with the virus. However all members of my household were vaccinated against the virus.

Hepatitis C Virus (HCV)

The Hepatitis C virus is often referred to as the dragon because it can stay in the body for a very long time without the individual *"The purpose of life is a life of purpose" Robert Byrne* knowing. The hepatitis C virus (HCV) was discovered in 1989 by workers at the Chiron Corporation, a biotechnology company. *"The current structure is derived from is got from structures of the proteins encoded by its genetic materials and compares to other related viruses. Its size is estimated by passing infected blood through filters." (Worman, 1999)* It was formally referred to as the "non-A, non-B" virus because people with hepatitis-like symptoms did not have the hepatitis A and B viruses in them. Since the 1970s, donated blood had been screened for the hepatitis A and B virus, and a lot of people still had hepatitis-like symptoms in the 1980s. They decided to call these groups of symptoms *non-A, non-B hepatitis* (NANB). In 1989, the CDC identified a separate virus that has hepatitis-like symptoms responsible for the NANB and called it Hepatitis C.

The hepatitis C virus is an RNA virus type called a *flavivirus*. It looks like the virus that causes yellow and dengue fever. The type of enzymes they produce characterizes them, and all show different clinical manifestations, genetic materials, and clinical prognosis.

How widespread is Hepatitis C?

- There are about 4 million people infected with the HCV virus in the USA and about 110 – 150 million people worldwide.
- There are about 36,000 new cases of HCV infection annually in the USA according to the CDC, and about 10,000 people die each year from hepatitis C.
- HCV accounts for one fifth of all acute viral hepatitis.
- Only about 25 percent of HCV-infected people are diagnosed annually.
- From 75 – 85 percent of HCV cases become chronic, and many infected people are unaware of their initial infection, sometimes for as long as 20 years after it occurred.
- HCV is one of the leading causes of liver transplantation in the U.S.
- Today, there is 1 in 600,000 chance of being infected from blood because of improvements on the blood supply system.
- The NIH has determined that 90 percent of hepatitis infections from blood transfusions are from the HCV.
- About 1 out of every 60 Americans has the HCV virus. The NIH estimates that today only 3 out of every 10,000 blood recipients contract the HCV virus.
- The American Liver Foundation estimates that the cost of treatment and management of HCV infection will rise to $85 billion dollars in the next 10 to 20 years if the illness is left unchecked.

What is your genotype?

The HCV virus, being a single-stranded RNA virus, can mutate into various subtypes because it does not have a repair mechanism to fix changes in its DNA. The genotype of HCV directly correlates with its path of infections, response against interferon and other treatments, its contagiousness, and the outcomes. Some subtypes are more virulent than others. There are six genetically-different variations of the HCV, called genotypes, and about 50 known subtypes of HCV. The type of enzymes they produce characterizes them, and they all show different clinical manifestations, different genetic materials, and different clinical prognoses.

- The genotypes 1a and 1b are more common in the U.S. They show more virulent clinical manifestations and progress with greater rapidity to liver cirrhosis, and they are also less likely to respond favorably to treatment with alpha interferon and Ribavirin.

- The majority of Americans have genotype 1a and 1b. This genotype is the hardest to manage and does not respond to interferon and combination therapy.
- The genotype subtype 1a is common in the U.S. and European countries. The subtype 1b is common in Japan and Europe. The genotype 1 is least responsive to conventional western treatments with interferon and Ribavirin.
- Genotype 2 is mostly found in Japan and China.
- Genotype 3 is mostly found in Scotland and other parts of the United Kingdom.
- Genotype 4 is mostly found in the Middle East and Africa.
- Genotype 5 is mostly found in Canada and South Africa.
- Genotype 6 is mostly found in Hong Kong and Macau.

How's HCV transmitted?

The HCV virus is a blood-borne virus i.e. it needs blood as a vehicle to move around the body

The US blood supply was contaminated with the HCV virus in the 1970s and 1980s because IV drug users donated or sold contaminated blood to blood banks. Similarly, Vietnam War veterans who were exposed to unsterile procedures and vaccinations during that war came home with the HCV virus. People who received the contaminated blood were subsequently involved with high-risk procedures that involved blood and the HCV epidemic got out of hand.

How does Acute and chronic HCV infection differ?

The determining factor that differentiates an acute episode from a chronic disease is the immunological state of the individual. Chronic hepatitis C indicates the presence of HCV RNA in the blood for more than six months. The HCV mutates very rapidly. This leads to *quasispecies* i.e. distinct but related genetic strains of the virus. People with the greatest numbers of quasispecies have the poorest response to interferon therapy and poorer prognosis. The longer the individual has HCV in her blood, the greater the number of quasispecies

Why do we have more cases of chronic hepatitis C than Hepatitis B?
Unlike hepatitis B, where only about 5 percent of infected people progress to the chronic stage, 85 percent of individuals infected with acute hepatitis C progress to the chronic phase. The reason is the presence of quasispecies of different traits of HCV virus. These variations collectively make them better armed to trick, elude, and fight the immune system. While the virus engages a particular mutant trait during the acute phase of the disease, the HCV virus often mutates to stronger and different traits referred to as quasispecies. This makes it able to outsmart the immune system, and particularly difficult for synthetic antivirals and interferons to eradicate it. (Palmer, 2004).

Doctors Heath Advisory: The HCV virus does not mutate against herbal antibiotics remedies.

Variables that affect the immunological state include the following:
- the age at which the infection was contracted
- the presence of venereal and other systemic diseases
- psychosomatic stress
- malnutrition
- lifestyles
- IV drug use and blood transfusions

What are the tests for HCV?
Blood tests determine the presence of hepatitis C antibodies (HCV Ab) in the blood in order to diagnose hepatitis C. The tests tell if the immune system is producing antibodies against the hepatitis C antigens. Diagnostic tests detect the presence of HCV antibodies in the blood, which indicates the presence of the virus in the blood. They also determine the extent of cell damage to the liver or detect elevation of liver enzymes as function of liver function.

Antibodies to the HCV virus are produced within the first 4 weeks of initial exposures to the virus in about 35 percent of individuals, while the remaining 65 percent develop antibodies 5 – 8 weeks after exposure to the virus. Unlike HIV, HCV is not routinely checked by doctors. Patients need to specifically ask their doctors for HCV test.

The **enzyme immunoassay test (EIA)** tests the presence of antibodies against the HCV, and has 96 percent sensitivity in chronic HCV individuals. EIA identifies the presence of antibodies to the HCV virus in about 85 percent of infected individuals at about 5 weeks after first exposure to the virus. The viral antibodies detected by this test do not confer immunity to infected people, and the EIA test does not distinguish between chronic and acute infection. It only detects the presence of the antibodies to the HCV virus in the blood. The test should be repeated to confirm the diagnosis. If the initial test is negative, the infection could have occurred within six months and the body may not have produced enough antibodies to the HCV virus to be detected in the blood. There may also be a lack of immunological response by the individual.

The **ELISA (Enzyme-linked immunosorbent assay) test** looks for the presence of antibodies in the blood against the HCV viral proteins. This is the first test routinely performed on chronic HCV patients for diagnostic purposes. It is also being used to screen donated blood. Blood that tests positive with ELISA is not allowed in blood banks. The positive ELISA test indicates chronic HCV pending definitive diagnosis. The ELISA test does establish exposure to the HCV but does not confirm if the infection is recent, past, or if the virus is eliminated from the blood. It also does not indicate the amount of antibodies in the blood. A more definitive test, the PCR test, provides more information. The ELISA test is negative for acute HCV infection because it takes more than six weeks for antibodies to show up from initial infection of HCV.

The **RIBA (Recombinant immmunoblot) assay confirms** the ELISA, and indicates which HCV antibodies are present. If it indicates the presence of only one antibody, the individual may or may not be infected. If it responds to two antibodies, there is definitely an infection with HCV. The RIBA assay rest does not measure the viral load.

What tests determine HCV viral load?
RNA assays, also called the HCV-RNA test, checks the viral load in the blood by targeting the viral RNA. This test will also indicate if the virus is active and multiplying in the blood stream.
The **PCR (Polymerase chain reaction)** test, also called RT-PCR tests, for the HCV RNA in the blood, i.e. the viral load per one milliliter of blood. It is used as a definitive diagnosis for the antibody tests, tracking response to treatment, and monitoring the viral load.

The **FDA-approved self test for HCV**, called the Home Access Hepatitis C Check Kit, came out in 1999. It is used to check for exposure to the HCV virus in the privacy of your home. For information on this test call 1-888-888-HEPC, or visit these websites: www.homeacess.com or www.homehealthtesting.com/hepatitis-c-tests.htm.

What happens when HCV infects the liver?

The HCV virus, like the Hepatitis B virus, has an affinity for the liver. It attacks the liver, takes over the host cell's nuclear DNA, and uses it as a template to multiply itself and produce more viruses. The host immune system responds accordingly by sending antibodies to arrest the situation and stop the ongoing viral multiplication. The instability of the HCV makes it hard for the immune system to get a firm grip on the virus, and as the virus eludes the white blood cells, the liver is often caught in a cat-and-mouse game between the virus and the immune system. The weapons directed at the virus by the immune system lands on the liver. The disruption of liver functions from these misdirected actions accounts for the initial acute symptoms of HCV.

Acute infection. During acute infections, nonspecific symptoms like malaise, abdominal pain, fatigue, nausea, and loss of appetite occur in about 20 percent of infected individuals. Individuals going through this phase feel weakened by the inflammatory process. The symptoms are mild, so most people do not seek medical help. The immune system overwhelms the virus, clears it from the body, and they are non-infective, do not get sick with the disease, and have lifelong immunity. For about 80 percent of people the damage is serious enough to weaken the immunological defenses which give rooms for viral proliferation. The white blood cells continuously make an effort to attack the virus in infected liver cells where the virus inculcates itself to replicate. A vicious cycle is established that is clinically referred to as the chronic phase of the disease.

Chronic infection If after six months of infection, the immune system has not rid the body of the virus; the disease is classified as chronic. About 46 percent of chronic carriers can live with the virus for 20 years and not know they are infected. They experience intermittent symptoms like fatigues, depression, memory problems, digestive problems, and muscles and joint aches. They are considered to be symptomatic carriers as they can spread the virus via blood or blood products. During this period, the virus continuously attacks the liver, and there is a constant struggle between the host's immune system and the virus. Symptoms of the infection may or may not be manifest, depending on the stresses and the immunological state of the infected individual. With time the virus infiltrates the blood supply to the liver. This is followed by death of the liver cells and could progress from fibrosis to cirrhosis and liver cancer.

How infective is the HCV?

- The HCV virus can live outside the body for about 4 – 6 hours and still be contagious.
- Unlike the HIV virus, HCV is not killed by bleach or chlorine disinfectants.
- It takes fewer viral particles to become infected with the HCV than with HIV. One single encounter is more likely to result in HCV infection than with the HIV virus. Unlike HIV virus, one single contact with infected blood can become a lifetime of infection.
- The HCV can survive in dried blood for about and three and one half months.

What lifestyles expose us to HCV?

Because HCV is a blood-born disease, infection can take place when we indulge in the following lifestyles or habits:

- Cocaine-snorting straws; microscopic droplets of blood are left on the straws from the nasal passages. Snorting cocaine irritates the nasal linings. The straws or rolled up papers used to sniff cocaine often pick up blood from the nostrils. When this used by another person, weeks or months later, people can be infected with the previous user's blood.
- Tattoos, acupuncture, pedicures, manicures, electrolysis, and body piercing; needles that are reused without proper sterilization constitutes the same risk as IV drug use. The best approach is to use disposable needles.
- Health care workers are exposed to blood on a regular basis through needle sticks and medical instruments.
- Shared personal items, e.g. razors, needles, manicures, toothbrushes, scissors, and clippers may carry blood residues which can be a means of transmission.

- Menstrual blood of infected women; the transmission of HCV during sex occurs when there is a tear in the tissue or skin of infected individuals. Monogamous sex is safer than with multiple partners. The risk of transmitting the HCV to a single long-term partner is very low. Relationships with people with more than one risk factor can increase the risk of infection.
- HCV is not transmitted through breastfeeding unless the nipples are cracked or bleeding, as the HCV virus need blood to be transmitted.
- High-risk homosexual and heterosexual behaviors increase the risk of transmission.
- Older people with reduced immunity are at risk of exposure.

You may already have HCV if you
- received blood transfusions during organ transplants or hemodyalysis before 1992;
- are a hemophiliac and received blood and clotting factors before 1987;
- Have had intimate relationships with someone infected with the HCV, including anybody with a history of multiple sex partners or STDs.
- have had tattoo or body piercing with tools that were not well sterilized;
- are a healthcare worker and have experienced needle sticks, cuts, or mucosal exposure;
- are a newborn or infant of an infected mother; or
- Have had dialysis with improperly sterilized instruments.

You cannot get HCV from
- any activity that does not involve transfer of blood;
- bodily fluids like saliva, urine, or semen;
- kissing or hugging;
- sharing household utensils;
- Sneezing or coughing; (HCV is not spread through the air i.e. it is not air borne.)
- Toilet seats.

What Happens If I have OTHER FORMS of Hepatitis and HIV WITH HCV?

- The presence of HAV, HBV, and HIV with HCV puts an extra burden on the liver and the immune system. Liver disease progresses more rapidly in individuals with HCV and other viral infections. The best approach is to manage the most serious of these diseases.
- After initial diagnosis of HCV, it is important to be vaccinated against HAV and HBV since about 5 percent of individuals with HCV and HIV have HBV.
- Individuals whose livers had been damaged by HCV cannot take protease inhibitors for their HIV infection because of its toxic effects on the liver. Individuals with HCV, HIV, and genotype 1a are more contagious and the illness progresses more rapidly because HCV and HIV drugs interact negatively and the cumulative effects of these viruses are too much for the immune system to handle.
- It is estimated that about 25 percent of people with both HIV and HCV do not produce antibodies to the HCV because the HIV had hampered their immune system and simple blood tests do not indicate HCV presence. This immuno-compromised state predisposes them to other types of hepatitis.
- It is recommended that people with HIV should be tested routinely for the presence of HCV co-infection.

Will my blood iron level affect HCV?

Studies show that there is correlation between iron intake and the inflammatory markers of patients with Hepatitis C. Just as the HCV virus have an affinity for the liver, it has an even stronger affinity for iron.

- HCV inflicts damage by latching onto iron stores in the liver. It causes free radical damage to liver cells. This sets the stage for inflammation and formation of scar tissue and cancer.
- High iron level is a contraindication for interferon therapy because high iron concentration in the liver reduces the efficacy of interferons. Reduction of iron levels in HCV patients is associated with normalization of liver enzymes and resolution of inflammation. It creates an unfavorable environment for the proliferation of the HCV.

- The failure of practitioners to embark on iron-depletion therapies before antiviral therapy accounts for high failure rates in the successful management of HCV infections.

Reducing your blood iron content naturally
- Restrict intake of iron-rich foods such as red meats, liver, iron-fortified cereals, and multivitamins. Avoid cooking with iron-coated cook wares and utensils.
- Lactoferrin, a sub-fraction of whey protein, has been shown to be a scavenger of free iron. Rubin (2002) indicates that homeostatic soil probiotic organisms contain substances that stimulate the formation of lactoferrin, a member of the iron-carrying protein family. The iron in lactoferrin is 95 percent bioavailable, but not to infectious pathogens.
- An alternative remedy that may facilitate the normalization of iron levels to the 30 – 80 mg/dL ranges includes high doses of green tea polyphenols and high-alicin garlic.
- High potency calcium supplements have also been shown to help reduce iron absorption by as much as 40 percent.

Why there is no vaccine against HCV
There is no vaccine for the HCV because the virus is very unstable. It changes its shape rapidly and mutates rapidly, changing its protein envelop to evade antibodies produced by vaccines.

Orthodox management of HCV
Interferons interfere with the replicative ability of HCV. An individual with chronic hepatitis does not produce enough interferons. If interferons are administered from exogenous sources, the liver might be able to fight the HCV virus and concurrently stimulate the host immune system.

The known types of interferons are alpha, beta, and gamma interferons, with the alpha most effective for the HCV virus. The body produces about 20 known types of alpha interferons and thousands of yet-to-be-discovered subtypes that a healthy leukocyte can produce. Synthetic alpha interferon is a needle in a hay stack when compared

"Like suicide bombers that self destruct to promote an ideology, Interferons are substances that make healthy- infected cells self destruct themselves as a nature's ways of stopping the spread of infections and preserving the host. The ideology of interferons is the survival of the individual host"

to the synergistic interactions needed for the interferons to launch an immunological response—a whole is greater than the sum of its parts.

Interferons were originally used to treat hairy-cell leukemia in 1986. The FDA approved its use for the management of HCV in 1991 to prevent the replication of HCV by empowering the immune system, reducing viral loads, slowing inflammation, addressing liver damage, and normalizing liver enzymes.

Who benefits from interferon therapy?

- Interferon therapy is only successful in about half of the patients treated. These groups of patient are called responders.
- The response to interferon usually occurs within the first eight weeks of treatment. It is often discontinued if the liver enzymes do not fall within normal range within three or four months of treatment.
- Most responders will relapse with elevated viral loads and liver enzymes if they discontinue taking interferon. This is often followed with Rebetron therapy, which ultimately restores normality.

What are the drawbacks of interferon therapy?

- Interferon reduces liver damage only in about 15 percent of HCV patients treated.
- About half of the people on interferon therapy do not respond to interferon at all.
- About 40 percent of those on interferon will see reduction in their viral loads to undetectable levels and normalized liver enzymes within the first six months.
- Anywhere from 8 – 20 percent of these patients can maintain these improvements for more than six months after interferon therapy is discontinued.
- People with HCV and undiagnosed co-infections with HBV do not respond favorably to interferon therapy because the HBV virus continues to multiply in the presence of interferon, and this does not stop the ongoing liver damage associated with interferon therapy.
- The HCV viral proteins are usually very unstable and continue to mutate and elicit resistance to interferon.

- Like pouring salt on a wound, interferon depresses the white blood cell count which further suppresses the immune system it was designed to stimulate.
- Interferon will cause thyroid imbalance which could become a permanent problem with prolonged use of interferon.
- Interferon cannot be used on pregnant women because of its unknown effect unborns.
- Interferon will not work on older people because of its deliberating side effects and their corresponding diminished immunity.
- It does not work well for African Americans partly because of their genotypes which is mostly genotype 1.
- By reducing platelets and neutrophil count in HCV patients who already have low platelets and neutrophil counts, interferons further compromise the body's ability to fight microbes and manufacture blood-clotting factors, which need to be enhanced in an ailing liver and which are necessary for the fight against the HCV virus.
- Interferons will exacerbate diabetes and thyroid disease.
- Interferon can cause potentially dangerous nervous and mental disorders which include depression, anxiety, and sleeplessness.
- Other adverse reactions include dry mouth, inflammation, and the possibility of infection at injection sites.
- Interferon is risky on people with the following conditions: bleeding, ascites, emotional problems, people taking immunosuppressive drugs, people with autoimmune diseases, and lung disease.
- The side effects of interferon includes flu-like symptoms like nausea, energy loss, fever, chills, muscle aches, irritability, depression, mild to moderate hair loss, diarrhea, sleeplessness, skin irritation, vertigo, and heart arrhythmia. About 25 percent of people who start on interferon drop out because of these unpleasant side effects. Conventionally, some of these adverse reactions are managed with acetaminophen and antidepressants which are very toxic to the liver.
- Interferon is not recommended for HCV-infected people with clinically de-compensated cirrhosis, i.e. livers that are

on the edge of failure. People who had received kidney or heart transplant and people with liver cancer.

Interferon-with-Ribavirin combination therapy

In combination therapy, Ribavirin is used with interferon to manage the HCV infection. Ribavirin is an antiviral, a nucleoside analogue which kills the virus by causing it to go into mutation overdrive (Cohen, Gish and Doner, 2001). Ribavirin is a synthetic compound originally approved for use as an aerosol against viral infections of the respiratory tract in children. The known side effects of Ribavirin include anemia, birth defects, hypertension, and chronic depression. It can find its way into the sperm and can be transmitted to a woman during intercourse to eventually cause birth defects. It is contraindicated in people with heart disease.

Ribavirin alone is ineffective against the HCV virus, but it is used in combination with interferon as the combination leads to reduction in viral load for up to 65 percent of its users. When Ribavirin is used in combination with interferon, it is only effective in about 35 percent of HCV patients.

While the management of HCV with interferon has adverse reactions, adding Ribavirin to the mix creates more adverse reactions as they are both synthetic products. It is believed that once treatment is stopped with HCV the virus often return in more virulent forms.

YOU CANNOT use interferon and/or Ribavirin IF
- you have de-compensated cirrhosis;
- you are an organ transplant recipient;
- you have depression, are taking antidepressants, or have suicidal tendencies; or
- You have not stopped taking alcohol or recreational drugs, have bone marrow disorders, and have HIV or anemia.

Reberton is also used in the management of hepatitis C, but has been shown to cause severe emotional disturbances, flu like symptoms, and birth defects.

Doctor's health advisory: Before starting any drug regimen, please ask your doctor for genotype testing. This is important because different genotypes react differently to medications.

IS THERE A CURE FOR HEPATITIS C?

Almost one in every 70 persons in the United States (that is 1.45% of the population) is estimated to be suffering from hepatitis C. For hepatitis C, cure is also known as 'Sustained Viral Remission' (SVR). According to a recent article published in June,2009 Hepatology, 'up to 50% of patients with chronic hepatitis C fail to respond to initial therapy with Pegylated Interferon(Peg-Ifn) and Ribavirin(RBV)'.With unsuccessful viral eradication, these individuals remain at risk for developing progression of their liver disease to cirrhosis and cancer. For individuals who are nonresponders, have low chances of hepatitis C sustained viral remission through conventional treatment or are frightened of the horrible side effects of hepatitis drugs, alternative remedies may be the needed hope. Hepatic herbs act on the hepato-biliary system. They act favorably on the liver and restore the deviated functioning back to normalcy. They reduce the viral count and activity by stimulating the immune system. They address the after effects of tissue changes due to the hepatitis C virus. They also work by stimulating the production of the antibodies, defence blood cells etc. In cases of immune disease, they seem to be working by correcting the immune mechanism. These hepatic herbs have been used successfully with a variety of results ranging from normalizing liver enzymes to total clearance and elimination of the hepatitis virus.

Hepatitis D Virus (HDV)

HDV is also called the hepatitis delta virus and belongs to the delta *viridae* family of viruses. It was first discovered in 1977 by Dr. Rizetto and his associates in Turin Italy. It requires the presence of hepatitis B for it to exist and multiply itself, since it cannot self-replicate. Its co-infection with HBV can lead to greater risk of liver failure. Its presence is indicated when HBV shows an increase and severity in acute symptoms. It becomes chronic as a super infection of HBV. About 75 – 80 percent of individuals with HBV and HDV develop liver cirrhosis compared with 15 – 30 percent of people with chronic HBV alone. HDV can cause acute and chronic hepatitis in people with HBV.

"There is only one corner of the universe you can be certain of improving and that is your own self"

Aldous Huxlety

Super infected individuals are people who are initially infected with HBV and later with HDV. HDV is commonly transmitted through blood and in people with history of IV drug use. It is diagnosed by blood testing for IgM and IgG antibodies. People with immunity against HBV cannot get infected with HDV so HBV vaccination is often a preventive against the HDV

Hepatitis E Virus (HEV)

It was originally referred to as energetically-transmitted non-A, non-B or water-borne, non-A, non-B hepatitis because it is mainly spread through water. The HEV is a member of the *caliciviridae* group of viruses. Hepatitis E like hepatitis A is spread through fecal-contaminated water and food. It always has acute symptoms and is identified only through lab tests. There are no specific treatments for the disease except for symptomatic treatments. It generally runs its course taking weeks or months. It is rare in the U.S. but common in developing countries.

"Ability is what you are capable of doing. Motivation determines what you do. .Attitude determines how well you do it"Lou Holtz

Hepatitis G (HGV)

This classification is given to individuals with chronic viral hepatitis that is not caused by Hepatitis B, C or the D viruses, cases of cirrhosis with unknown etiology and other forms of hepatocellular carcinoma. Polymerase Chain reaction tests (PCR) indicate the presence of this virus. It is seen among healthy blood donors. It does not worsen pre existing liver disease

Non-Infectious Causes of Liver Diseases

Non-contagious hepatitis stems from prescription and non-prescription drugs, poisons, alcohol, chemicals, food, water, and environmental pollutants which are classified as toxins. Since many of these are not part of the natural ecosystem, human livers are not adapted to metabolize them. They create metabolic challenges to the liver.

How does alcohol affect my liver?

Excessive use of alcohol is very detrimental to the immune system and the liver, and predisposes humans to a wide variety of immunological disorders. Alcohol has a strong ability to weaken the immune system. Only about 6 percent of the alcohol consumed is eliminated from the body via the urine, the lungs, and the sweat glands. The remainder is oxidized in the liver into very toxic end products like aldehydes and carbon dioxide.

Alcohol metabolism blocks the assimilation and synthesis of essential nutrients by the liver. Being devoid of any nutrient, it is classified as a foodless or empty carbohydrate. This creates the illusion of energy and fullness hence people who consume alcohol regularly don't have urge to eat. This is the reason why alcoholics are malnourished. This decreased appetite associated with alcohol consumption robs the body of the needed nutrients, especially a compromised liver. Acetaldehyde exerts its toxic effect on the liver by inhibiting cellular mitochondria functions and reactions.

Alcohol binds to a variety of proteins and alters liver functions and structure, thereby making the liver cells (hepatocytes) swell which causes a fatty liver. If this is not treated, it progresses to alcoholic hepatitis and cirrhosis, which accounts for about 25 percent of mortalities associated with alcoholism. Alcohol also impairs enzymatic activities and vitamin activation. Alcohol is metabolized in the liver by the cytochrome P450 enzymes. Some drugs that are metabolized by these enzyme systems compete with alcohol for their metabolism. This creates an unnecessary back up of toxic metabolites in the body. This is what leads to severe injuries associated with drug and alcohol interactions. When drugs are held up in the body for longer periods, they react with other substances to form toxic intermediates substances that can have potentially fatal adverse reactions.

Those who choose to consume alcohol should avoid acetaminophen up to 24 hours after the consumption of alcohol. Heavy alcohol drinkers are not eligible for liver transplants, and alcohol use reduces their life span by about 10 years. Government does not regulate the processing of alcohols and the herbs used to make alcoholic beverages. The pesticides in alcoholic beverages and the aluminum cans in which they are packaged constitute a double jeopardy to the human immune system.

How does tobacco affect my liver?
Tobacco leaves are grown under unregulated deplorable soil conditions with insecticides, pesticides, fungicides, and preservatives. There are over 60 known cancer-causing chemicals in tobacco smoke. Nicotine is classified as a scheduled poison under the Therapeutic Good Act. In addition to nicotine, smokers also inhale about 4,000 other chemicals. Tobacco smoke

also contains tar, carbon monoxide, hydrogen cyanide, free radicals, lead, arsenic, cadmium, and radioactive compounds. Normally, oxygen is transported to the various organs in the body by binding to hemoglobin, a red blood cell protein. Carbon monoxide is an odorless gas that is fatal in large quantities. Carbon monoxide displaces oxygen in the blood because it has a greater affinity for hemoglobin than oxygen. Carbon monoxide is readily carried to the organs and tissues by attachment to hemoglobin instead of oxygen. Consequently, the liver and other organ tissues in the body are deprived of much-needed oxygen because of carbon monoxide from tobacco smoke. The reduction of oxygen flow to the liver hampers its cellular activities.

How do prescription drugs affect the liver?

Every drug affects a natural enzyme system within the body to treat conditions. Most of the time, they complete the process successfully. Problems arise when the same drug affects other enzyme systems in harmful ways. It is impossible to predict all possible side effects of any particular drug. It is also impossible for doctors and pharmacist to predict the path of any drug. This unpredictability is what causes the problems associated with drug use. "In-vivo" does not always translate to "in-vitro". The liver is the organ that detoxifies all the drugs we consume. Each drug uses one particular enzyme system for its metabolism. Bottlenecks hold ups, and backups occur in the liver when more than one drug is consumed that utilizes the same enzyme system. Consequently, these drugs stay in the body longer and climb to dangerous levels. Drug metabolism creates intermediate toxic by products in the body before being eliminated. The liver may then have to change a drug chemically more than one time into a product the body can excrete. These products can often be more toxic than the actual drug itself, especially if there is a hold up. These processes put a lot of strain on the liver. It is the toxic consequences of these drugs, their intermediate by-products, and the cumulative side effects that constitute disruption of liver functions referred to as drugs-induced or toxic hepatitis.

The grim statistics of prescription drug use in the United States

- Over-the-counter medications cause an average of 16,000 deaths per year in the United States (Strand, 2003).
- Ninety-eight percent of all prescription and non-prescription drugs precipitate constitutional acidity in which viruses thrive. (Baroody, 2001).
- Thirty-six million prescription for pain killers and 275 billion prescriptions for antibiotics are filled annually in the United States. (Holford, 1999)
- Adverse drug reactions are the third leading causes of deaths in the U.S. after heart disease and cancer. Drug induced illnesses (e.g. drug-induced hepatitis) are often caused by these adverse reactions which are mistaken for new diseases, requiring new prescriptions and constituting a vicious circle of prescription drug use. Strand (2003).
- Before 1990, only 3 – 4 percent of new drugs were first released in the U.S., but today 66 percent of all new drugs released are first approved and released in the U.S. (Strand, 2003).

- According to the Kaiser Family Foundation, drug companies are reaping four dollars in profit for every one dollar spent on drug ads, and *Reuters Business Insight*, a publication for investors, observes that the future of the industry depends on its ability to "create new disease markets." These markets are designed to sell a problem and not the solution.
- According to the General Accounting Office, drug companies spent four billion dollars in advertising, and only one-seventh of that amount was spent on research and development. These advertisements drive up health care costs in the United States and seduce millions into asking their doctors for drugs for disease they have never heard of. These practices leads patients to self diagnose and ignore lifestyle changes that may be more beneficial than drugs.

Why we don't get healed in the Hospital

The motto of the teaching hospitals of most universities is "we care, God heals". Excellent care is rendered in the hospitals, but the healing essence of nature is absent.

"God heals and the doctor gets paid"
Benjamin Franklin

Healing is a different thing altogether from the care rendered. Unless we carry our health above the standard of care obtained in the hospital environment, we can never be healed or become whole again. The hospital environment is too synthetic and artificial for healing to take place. *Healing is not scientific but an intuitive art of wooing nature to serve us. Only nature can heal that which it has made.*

Every body is inhaling air exhaled by other sick people. The most serious failure of the hospital is in malnutrition. Dietary regimens of the wrong foods and deficiencies of healing foods predominate the hospital menu. The lymphatic and circulatory system must flow like a river to have optimum absorption of nutrients and elimination of toxins. In the hospital, there is attendant stagnation. Stagnation, automation, and sedentary life breeds degeneration.

Originally, the word hospital is derived from the root word "hospice", meaning a place to die (Brooner Jr., 2000). Doctor's care, palliative care, medicines, and exploratory surgeries should be adjuncts to wholeness through natural endowments like fresh air, sunlight, purified water, whole foods, and softening of attitudes. Because these conditions do not exist in the hospital environment, we do not get healed. The hospital environment subdues, rather than working with nature. Fluorinated and chlorinated tap water are given to patients in most hospitals, and meals are improperly prepared. The very foods and food combinations that cause people to be admitted to the hospital are served in the hospital. Over 95 percent of the meals served in the hospital are not organically grown, despite the overwhelming evidence that correlates processed foods, pesticides, insecticides and herbicides with chronic degenerative diseases.

⊠ *Flashback*
It has been three months since I was admitted to the hospital, and the interventional care I received was pivotal to my being alive today. For me to bet healed of my condition, I needed to be out of the synthetic environment and off of drugs. I contracted a life-threatening bacterial infection in the hospital that was unresponsive to the antibiotic I was administered. I had to be rushed out of the hospital like I was rushed in and provided with a home healthcare nurse to administer the antibiotic Ciprofloxacin to me intravenously. This provided me the opportunity to experience nature. When I came back to the hospital after I stabilized, I found that two of the residents had committed

suicide from job-related stress. Studies show that patients are ten times more likely to acquire infections in the hospital that out of the hospital. Infections acquired in the hospital are called nosacomial infections.

The grim statatistics
- Nationally, the average patient receives about 10 different drugs on admission to the hospital, while those who are critically ill receive an average of about 38 different medications. (Strand, 2003)
- About 15 percent of patients admitted to hospitals suffer from adverse drug reactions. (Strand, 2003).
- Adverse drug reaction is five times more likely to kill than being in an automobile or AIDS. (Strand, 2003).

What is autoimmune Hepatitis?
In autoimmune diseases, our immune system, designed to protect us against external invasion, becomes our foe. The antibodies in the blood are attacking the fats, tissues, organs, or DNA inside our cells. Like an automobile operating with adulterated fuels, immune dysfunctions are common in our chemically-overloaded environment. Gilbert (2006) stresses that growing numbers of autoimmune and inflammatory diseases are attributed to causes within the body and its surroundings. When the human body is overloaded with toxins, the immune system becomes overloaded and irritated. Consequently, it responds to these toxins with excess inflammatory chemicals and antibodies because the immune system is in a hyper-stimulated state.

"If one advances confidently in the direction of his dreams and endeavors to live the life which he has imagined, he will meet with success unexpected in common hour"
Henry David Thoreau

This often leads to a wide variety of immune-related illnesses, like swollen glands, recurrent infections, chronic-fatigue syndrome, fibromyalgia, systemic lupus, rheumatoid arthritis, primary biliary cirrhosis, vasculitis, sclerosing cholangitis, sarcoid, multiple sclerosis, lupus erythematosus, thyroiditis, ulcerative colitis, vitiligo (loss of skin pigmentation), and sjorgrens syndrome that is characterized by dry eyes and dry mouth.

With regard to food allergies from wheat, corn, and dairy and their relation to autoimmune illnesses, the circulating immune complexes, or CICs, start out as extra-large protein molecules that are only partially digested in the small intestine and before being absorbed into the bloodstream. Once in the bloodstream, the immune system treats them as invaders because they are too large to be metabolized, provoking an immune reaction. Antibodies couple with these foreign protein invaders to form CICs. At first, these CICs may be neutralized in the lymphatic system. But over time, as more CICs are created, they overwhelm the body's ability to eliminate them. They overwhelm the immune system and the kidneys. At that point, the body has no choice but to "store" them in its soft tissues, where the immune system continues to attack them as allergens causing inflammation and, ultimately, autoimmune disorders.

Conventional medicine responds to autoimmune diseases with suppressive steroids (e.g. prednisone and azathioprine) which further exacerbate the toxic load of the immune system and push hyper-stimulation over the top. These steroids arrest hyper-stimulation by suppressing the immune responses to exogenous or endogenous inducers. Adversely, they lower the overall immune system response and expose humans to wide varieties of contagious diseases. In autoimmune hepatitis, the hyper-stimulated antibodies of the immune system are attacking the liver cells (hepatocytes). Autoimmune hepatitis is associated with an increase in circulating antinuclear antibodies and gamma globulin which leads to inflammations in the liver. In other autoimmune diseases of the liver like primary biliary cirrhosis, the immunological cells attack the smallest bile ducts in the liver, causing obstruction and inflammation.

Serum protein electrophoresis and immunological testing are used to diagnose autoimmune hepatitis. Patients with auto immune hepatitis develop cirrhosis and will eventually require liver transplants despite the use of steroids in management of cirrhosis. Steroid prescriptions for patients with autoimmune hepatitis usually results in weight gain. In such situations, it is advisable to use a varied and well-balanced diet.

Managing Autoimmune Hepatitis
If weight gain from prescription steroids is excessive, it is advisable to reduce foods high in calories. These foods include sweets, sugars, cakes, biscuits, fried foods, pies, crisps, and chocolates. Low-fat versions of these foods are advised. Immunological testing for the presence of anti-mitrochrondial and antinuclear antibodies and liver biopsy are used in the diagnosis of primary

biliary cirrhosis. Bile acids like ursodiol are used in the management of primary biliary cirrhosis. The disease eventually progress to the need for a liver transplant.

Complimentary alternative remedies for autoimmune Hepatitis
- The first rule in alternative medicine is to remove the probable-cause toxins.
- Eliminate all recreational drugs and risky lifestyles like alcohol and tobacco use, environmental allergies, irritants, and paying close attention to the water, food, medicines, and chemicals in the work and home environment. This is usually very beneficial in removing exogenous causes and halting the progression of the illness. I recommend replacing cow's milk with any of the following: organic rice milk, organic goat milk, or soy milk. Organic foods, filtered water, free-range poultry, grass-fed meats, and wild-caught sea foods.
- Heavy metal detoxification with organic juicing and chelation therapy are highly recommended for individuals with autoimmune diseases and autoimmune hepatitis. This helps to eliminate probable endogenous causes.
- Other detoxification therapies include colonics, enemas, foot detox, and infrared saunas.
- Eliminate psychosomatic stress.

Other liver diseases
Primary Sclerosing Cholangitis (PSC)
In primary sclerosing cholangitis (PSC), the immune system turns itself on the larger bile ducts inside and outside the liver and elicits symptoms similar to the obstruction of the bile ducts. It is associated ulcerative colitis i.e. inflammatory bowel disease. The resulting inflammation causes obstruction to the flow of bile, obstruction of the bile ducts with the liver, biliary cirrhosis, frequent episodes of bacterial cholangitis, and cancer of the bile ducts. This adversely affects *"Human beings can alter their* digestion of fats and fat-soluble vitamins *liver by altering their attitudes"* (e.g. A, D, E, and K) in the intestine as *William James* the supply of bile is reduced. Individuals develop a type of diarrhea which causes bulky, pale feces that is difficult to flush, nausea, and a general bloated feeling. A low-fat diet will help reduce this fatty diarrhea. The diagnosis of primary sclerosing cholangitis

is made when the presence of elevated alkaline phosphate and GGTP and bile obstructions or bacterial cholangitis occurs (Worman, 1999). Approximately 35 percent of PSC patients have an elevated gamma-globulin concentration in the blood, approximately 55 percent of PSC patients have elevated total blood IgM concentrations, and approximately 50 percent of patients with PSC have anti-neutrophilcytoplasmic antibodies. The diagnosis of PSC is made with endoscopic retrograde cholangiopancreatography (ERCP).There are no clear cut remedies for this disease. It eventually progresses to end stage cirrhosis requiring liver transplantation (Worman, 1999)

Primary Biliary Cirrhosis

Primary Biliary Cirrhosis (PBC) is one of the cholestatic liver diseases characterized by inflammation of the intra-hepatic bile ducts i.e. within the liver. It is characterized as a chronic lifelong illness with an autoimmune component. The cells lining the bile ducts in the liver are attacked by the body's own immune system in PBC damaging the bile ducts and spilling out bile acids. Because bile acids are strong detergents, they can damage and scar the liver tissues, causing cirrhosis; hence it is called biliary cirrhosis (Palmer, 2004). Some individuals may never progress to cirrhosis. If it causes complete disruption of bile flow, it is referred to as intra-hepatic cholestasis. It occurs mostly in middle-aged women. It gradually progresses to cirrhosis as it presents few or no symptoms. It is diagnosed from biopsies, immunological tests, and histological and laboratory evaluations. It causes elevated liver enzymes.

What are the symptoms of PBC?

- About 60 percent of people with PBC show no symptoms.
- chronic fatigue
- itching
- emotional disturbances
- sleep disorders
- unexplained weight loss
- enlarged liver and spleen
- fatty yellow nodules or patches on the skin called xanthalasma and xanthoma
- severe scratches with breaks in the skin, referred to as excoriations
- Individuals with PBC may experience hearth burn and an unpleasant acid taste in the mouth caused by the effects of

stomach acid. This is managed by avoiding eating late at night or raising the head of the bed by four or five inches.

Diagnosing PBC
PBC is diagnosed with a combination of physical exams, biopsy, radiological tests, and blood work. It is conventionally managed with ursodiol (Actigall™), a bile acid (Worman, 1999).

Wilson Disease
Wilson disease occurs when the liver's ability to synthesize copper is hampered. Consequently, excess copper accumulates in major organs like the cornea, liver, brain, and other organs in the body. Cooper overload causes behavioral disorders, unsteady gait, depression, and suicidal ideation, loss of mental functions, neurological disorders, osteoporosis, hemolytic anemia, and kidney damage. It causes damage to all the major organs where it accumulates. In the eye cornea, Wilson disease is characterized by brown pigments referred to as Kayser-Fleisher rings. The first line of management of the disease is the avoid foods high in copper like shellfish, mushrooms, liver, chocolate, and nuts.

Wilson disease is managed with chelating agents like Trientine and D-penicillamine, which pull excess copper from tissues. Supervised use of zinc as a dietary supplement helps remove copper from the body. An alternative approach to the management of Wilson disease involves heavy-metal detoxification programs that employ chlorophyll-rich plants like chlorella. Chlorophyll is very crucial in the elimination of heavy metals from the body.

Hemochromatosis (iron) Overload
Hemochromatosis is a genetic disease that causes excessive absorption of iron from food. This condition manifests itself as deficiencies in the body's ability to assimilate iron and to respond to iron overload, allowing excess iron to accumulate in the tissues. A disease of iron metabolism manifests itself by the deposition of excess iron in the body, which disrupts the functions of affected organ systems, causing decreased body hair, reduced interest in sex, weakness, fatigue, weight loss, liver pain, enlarged liver, enlarged heart, hyper pigmentation of the skin (bronze skin tone), diabetes, arthritis,

"Opportunity is missed by most people because it is dressed in overall and looks like work" Thomas Edison

impotence in men, lack of menstruation in women, and a variety of non-specific symptoms. Because of the non-specific symptoms associated with the disease, people go undiagnosed for a long time. Another reason people do not get early diagnosis is because of blood loss from regular blood donations, multiple pregnancies, menstruation, and gastrointestinal bleeding. The American Iron Overload Disease Association recommends regular screening for iron overload in all Americans 18 years and older. Since it takes a long time for iron to accumulate and cause its damage, symptoms are not noticed until the late stages of the illness. The disease is more prominent in men than women because women loss some iron monthly during menstruation.

Iron-induced oxidation of the liver-cell walls is called lipid peroxidation. The by-products of lipid peroxidation, like hydrogen peroxide, causes toxic harm to the hepatocytes liver cells. It occurs from free radical damage to fat cells. The cell membranes consist mainly of fatty layers of phospholipids which are compromised by oxidative stress. When the membranes are stressed, the genetic materials are compromised and internal organelles leak out. This also affects circulating lipids in the body that includes cholesterol, of which 85 percent is produced by the liver. The standard American diet has excessive amounts of iron that far exceed iron loss due to break down of hemoglobulin and during menstruation. Excess iron is stored in the liver as ferritin.

How is iron overload treated?
Hemochromatosis is less common among women due to blood loss from menstruation and pregnancy. High levels of iron in the human body are associated with increased risk of cirrhosis. Since the hepatitis C virus needs iron to replicate, alternative remedies can be employed to compliment conventional blood letting to reduce the iron load.

- The first line of management of hemochromatosis is avoidance of red meat, iron utensils and cookware, and iron-fortified foods.
- Synthetic amino acids, given intravenously, bind and extract heavy metals from the body.
- Complimentary alternative remedies achieve heavy-metal detoxification with chelating agents.

Fatty Liver: Non-Alcoholic Liver Disease (NALD)

Fatty liver (steatosis) is a disease associated with accumulation of fats in the liver cells. It is related to exposures to environmental toxins, drug use, alcoholism, obesity, and degenerative diseases. Cirrhotic livers cannot *"Right temporarily defeated is stronger than evil triumphant"MLK Jr.* process fat, and the liver cells cannot process cholesterol because of their inability to synthesize lipoproteins needed for cholesterol synthesis and transport. Consequently cholesterol level drops. The inability of cirrhotic livers to process fats make for the excretion of fats in the stools called steatorrhea. This is characterized by light colored stool.

Most toxins are fat-soluble and when the detoxification mechanism breaks down, accumulated toxins are stored in the cell membranes of cells which include liver cells. The accumulation of fat in the liver cells hampers their efficiency. This progresses to cell death through fibrosis (steatohepatitis) to cirrhosis.

Other Causes of Fatty Liver:
- Consuming too much fat, greasy food and unhealthy dietary lifestyles
- Drinking too much alcohol
- Not getting enough exercise
- Excessive weight
- Insulin resistance

What are the Remedies for Fatty Liver?
- Individuals are advised to do more exercise like walking or swimming.
- Eat plenty of fruits or vegetables.
- Eat more slow-release starchy foods (complex carbohydrates).
- Avoid refined sugars and starch.
- Lower weight to a healthy level.
- Substitute hydrogenated oils with healthy fats that are rich in essential fatty acids

Fatty liver is usually diagnosed with radiological tests, liver biopsy, and blood tests.

"Nothing in life is to be feared, it is only to be understood"
Marie Curie

Cholesterol and Liver Disease

Cholesterol is a waxy substance found in the blood stream and the cell membranes of the body's cells. Ordinarily, it is essential for a variety of functions in the body, and when its level gets too high, it becomes a risk factor in heart disease.

Cholesterol is derived from two main sources:
- From the body; the liver manufactures most of the body's cholesterol.
- From animals like meat, poultry, fish, sea foods, and dairy products (about 15 percent)

Plant foods do not contain cholesterol. What differentiates fats from cholesterol is that dietary fats consist of fatty acids, made from carbon, hydrogen and oxygen, that may be saturated, monounsaturated, or polyunsaturated. They are added to food to elicit taste and texture.

Saturated fats are derived from tropical oils like coconut oil and palm oil, and animal sources like butter, meat, lard, and whole-meat products. They are solid at room temperatures. Saturated fats from animal sources raise blood cholesterol and increase the risk for heart disease, while those from unprocessed tropical oils do not raise blood cholesterol.

Polyunsaturated fats come from botanical sources like safflower oils, corn, and soy. They are liquid at room temperature and are good sources of omega-3 and omega-6 fatty acids. When they are unrefined, the help lower blood cholesterol. They are found mainly in fish, especially salmon, green leafy vegetables, and flax seeds and oil. They do not raise blood cholesterol.

Monounsaturated fats are derived from botanical sources like olive oil, canola oil, peanut oil, sesame oil, avocado, walnut oils, and pumpkin. They are liquid at room temperature, and reduce bad cholesterol without affecting good cholesterol levels.

Hydrogenated or *partially-hydrogenated fats*, also referred to as trans-fats, are processed polyunsaturated fats. They are chemically altered to ensure chemical stability and longer shelf life in stores. They are used in restaurants, fast-food restaurants, and sold as vegetable oils. They raise the level of bad cholesterol. They are commonly used to prepare baked foods, packaged food, margarine, shortenings, cookies, crackers, peanut butter, and deep-fried foods to add texture and taste. They are a manufacturer's delight, but they are detrimental to human health.

Cholesterol is manufactured in the liver and transported through the blood stream by a group of proteins manufactured by the liver called lipoproteins. The blood, being mainly water, has to latch on to these lipoproteins to travel successfully around the body.

The *low-density lipoproteins* (LDL) are major transporters of cholesterol from the liver to the organs of the body. LDL is termed "bad cholesterol" because it carries excess oxidized cholesterol in the circulatory system to be deposited in arteries where it can cause reduced blood flow to the heart and vital organs like the brain, causing heart attacks and strokes.

High-density lipoproteins (HDL) are proteins that are also manufactured in the liver. They are called "good cholesterol" because it carries excess unneeded cholesterol away from the arteries to the liver where it is broken down into bile acids and excreted out of the body.

The LDL and HDL function as a two-way traffic system that transports cholesterol to and from the liver. Individuals whose livers manufacture low LDL and high HDL have a lower risk of developing coronary artery diseases. Conversely, individuals with low HDL and high LDL have a higher risk of developing coronary artery diseases.

☒ *Flashback*
For my astronomically-high LDL and triglycerides cholesterol, I was prescribed a statin drug, Zocor, with which elevated liver enzyme levels is a contraindication. The cocktail of chemotherapy and cholestero- lowering drugs pushed me to the frontiers of drug-induced (toxic) hepatitis. My blood level of LDL (low density cholesterol) indicates the probability of plaques building in my arteries, impeded blood flow to my extremities, kidney, brain, and heart. While my doctors believed my elevated cholesterol level was genetic, I demurred with the following explanations. The gene-disease theory stems from the work of Charles Darwin who in the twilight of his life recounted these concepts with the following statements "In my opinion, the greatest error which I have committed has been not allowing sufficient weight to the direct action of the environments, i.e. food, climate etc. independently of natural selection...when I wrote "The

origin", and for some years afterwards, I could find little good evidence of direct action of the environment; now there is a large body of evidence". While the originator of the gene theory of disease believes genes don't determine our destiny, conventional medicine needs this theory to propagate disease care over health i.e. to emphasize the problem over the person.

Misinformation about Cholesterol: Barking up the wrong tree

Cholesterol seals blood vessels and prevents leakage of blood. Blaming cholesterol for heart attacks and heart disease is like blaming the tire shop for your flat tire. When the doctor says you have high blood cholesterol, she is only measuring your arterial blood cholesterol. If cholesterol in the arterial blood causes heart disease, why doesn't cholesterol build up in the veins when the same blood flows through both vessels? The difference is because of the presence of muscle tissues that help sustain blood pressures in the arteries that are absent in veins.

When humans consume excessive amounts of saturated fats from animal sources, fried foods, simple carbohydrates, hydrogenated oils, and processed foods, those fats build up as toxic deposits in the arterial blood vessels and in fatty tissues of the body, increasing inflammations and damage to the blood vessels. Sedentary lifestyles, cigarette smoking, and lack of exercise also contribute to high blood cholesterol. As you will see, the inflammatory reactions generated from these habits and lifestyles destroy the integrity of the blood vessels and make them prone to leakage and breakage as the body becomes more acidic. Once body fluids becomes acidic, lactic acid degeneration translates into inflammations on the arterial muscular surfaces. Muscle tissues in arteries are more susceptible to disintegration by lactic acid, since the acidic body fluids dissolving the muscles, making then thin and weak. It is these inflammations of the muscular tissues of blood vessels that cause heart attacks, not cholesterol. These views are congruent with the those expressed in the April 1997 issue of the New England Journal of Medicine that suggest that cholesterol is not the primary cause of heart disease but inflammations of the blood vessels. With disintegrated muscular tissues, arterial walls are thinned, weakened, and becomes susceptible to breaks and leaks that translates as impending heart attacks (Barefoot, 2002).

To prevent heart attacks, the body develops compensatory mechanisms by attracting a variety of substances like the LDL cholesterols as reinforcements for the venerable arterial sites. The presences of cholesterol at these break-prone sites are protective and preventive mechanisms developed by nature to prevent impending breaks that would have resulted in death. This is like sealing leaks in your plumbing system or fixing a flat tire. These reinforcements make arterial walls thick, hard, and narrow. Rather than addressing the underlying causes from a nutritional viewpoint, conventional medicine blames family genes, all the while translating these occurrences as heart disease and as an indicator for the use of statin drugs, a multibillion dollar bonanza. Once again the care of the disease has taken precedence over the care of the individual.

When the cholesterol lowering drugs fail to lower blood cholesterol conventional medicine resorts to different surgical procedures like balloon angiography, surgical removal of plaques, and bypass surgeries that treats the disease and bypass the problem—malnutrition, acidosis and western diets.

How does the body produce cholesterol?
Cholesterol is actually a by-product produced while the body is synthesizing a little known substance called *mevalonate*. Mevalonate help control vascular tone and systemic blood pressure. Mevalonate synthesis is orchestrated by the enzyme HMG-CoA reductase. Cholesterol lowering drugs work by inhibiting this enzyme, hence they are called HMG-CoA reductase inhibitors. When doctors use statin drugs to inhibit the mevalonate pathway, they inhibits its function like maintaining blood pressure and vascular tone. Ironically cholesterol is not the only product of the Mevalonate chain that is inhibited by cholesterol lowering drugs. Other end products disrupted include co-enzyme Q10 and dilochol.

Co-enzyme Q10 is found in all cell membranes where it maintains cellular integrity and nerve functions. It is vital to the formation of elastin and collagen. The disruption of co-enzyme Q10 by statin drugs leads to weak heart muscles and the attendant increase in heart-failure rate associated with cholesterol lowering drugs. This explains why people on statin drugs have muscle pain, joint pain and failure of the heart muscle.

⊠ *Flashback*

The disruption of this important intermediate (Co-enzyme Q10) by Zocor™ accounts for the serious side effects I experienced, like severe back pain, muscle and joint pain, neuropathy, and inflammation of the tendons and ligaments. I am one of the lucky few saved from heart failure which is a major side effect of Zocor's blocking of co-enzyme Q10 synthesis.

The decision of drug companies to block the synthesis of mevalonate is because reduced amounts of mevalonate make smooth muscles less active and platelets less able to produce clots that can cause a heart attack. This explains why drug companies market statin drugs as preventing heart attacks. The risks of heart attacks and death are reduced but not eliminated because cholesterol is just one of the multitude of risk factors associated with heart attacks. While the incidence of heart attacks is reduced in the short term, there is a dramatic increase in the number of heart-failure cases caused by co-enzyme Q10 inhibition with these drugs.

High blood cholesterol exhibited no external signs or symptoms until doctors studied how to evaluate blood levels of cholesterol and used unrealistic indices to determine what is normal and what is abnormal. The bar kept being lowered to include perfectly healthy people whose only offence was having high cholesterol. About 26 years ago, the parameter was any middle-aged man whose cholesterol is over 240 with associated risk factors like smoking and being overweight. After the 1984 cholesterol consensus conference, the dragnet was expanded to include anyone, male or female, with cholesterol over 200 as candidates for statin drugs. Recently, the bar was lowered further to include anyone with cholesterol over 180. Currently, the qualifiers are extended to include individuals who suffered a heart attack even if their blood cholesterol is already very low. Current standards stipulate cholesterol evaluations and treatment for young adults and children. The beneficiaries of these are the drug companies and the casualties are the people needlessly suffering from heart failure, bypass surgery, and untold numbers undergoing balloon angioplasty and adverse reactions to statin drugs.

Functions of Cholesterol
- All cell membranes in the human body contain cholesterol. It makes the cells waterproof. The cells will be porous and leak without cholesterol.

- Cholesterol is the body's repair substance, as scar tissues contain high levels of cholesterol, including the arterial scar tissues.
- Cholesterol is a precursor to vitamin D. Bile salts needed for digestion of fats are made from cholesterol, and people with low cholesterol have difficulty digesting fats.
- Cholesterol plays an important role in the formation of brain matter. It is the main organic molecule of the brain and half of the dry weight of the cerebral cortex. It is responsible for the uptake of serotonin. When cholesterol levels are low, serotonin receptors do not work.
- Cholesterol is the precursor to all hormones produced in the adrenal cortex. This includes the glucocorticoids, which regulate the blood-sugar levels and mineral corticoids which regulate mineral balance. It promotes healing and balances tendencies towards inflammation. Cholesterol lowering drugs can disrupt the activity of the adrenal hormones.

Before the Statin Drugs
Statins replaced drugs that reduced blood cholesterol by disrupting its absorption in the intestines. The side effects of these drugs were unbearable and included constipation, nausea, and indigestion. They did not have any significant effect on blood cholesterol.

In 1958, Dr. Lester M. Morrison, the director of a research unit at Los Angeles County General Hospital published some findings in the January 1959 number of *Geriatrics* on the efficacy of lecithin in lowering blood cholesterol levels. He indicated that lecithin caused a 41 percent reduction in blood cholesterol in 80 percent of his patients suffering from high serum cholesterol levels. He indicated that lecithin facilitated their metabolism in the digestive tract and facilitated their transport through the vasculo-circulatory system. By emulsifying fats and cholesterol in the diet into tiny particles and holding them in suspension, lecithin prevented them from clumping together and sticking to blood platelets or the walls of the blood vessels. It is when dietary fats are not well emulsified that they stick together, form blood clots, and block arteries.

The word lecithin is derived from the Greek word for "egg yolk" where it was first isolated in 1850 by Maurice Bobley. Egg yolk is an excellent source of lecithin. Lecithin derived from animal sources are less active than those derived from plant sources. Obtained from soybeans, lecithin helps in the re-absorption of cholesterol back into the blood stream that has adhered to the walls of blood vessels. Lecithin derived from animal sources have higher levels of saturated fatty acids, while those derived from vegetable sources have higher levels of unsaturated fatty acids. Lecithin is essential in transporting triglycerides out of the liver, which prevents fatty liver. Most liver metabolism occurs in the membranes and this is where lecithin comes into play. Lecithin is mainly composed of choline and inositol, both of which are required for the breakdown of cholesterol. The choline is subsequently converted to acetylcholine. Many people take lecithin for it's choline component. Lecithin emulsifies fats into absorbable droplets like solvents cutting down grease. As an excellent emulsifier, it increases the bioavailability of nutrients with which it is co-administered.

Normally oil and water do not mix, but lecithin holds them together and keeps them from separating out. Thus, it helps to remove fatty deposits from the liver so they are unable to settle and form dangerous deposits. It helps prevent accumulation of deposits in arteries and melts those already present.

Phosphotidylcholine (PC) is a lecithin derivative obtained from soy lecithin. Lecithin granules are rich sources of phosphatidylcholine. Phosphatidylcholine is a major component of liver cellular membranes. PC is the universal building block for cell membranes, and the majority of metabolic activities that occur in the liver and most organs in the human body occur in the cell membranes. Since the damage caused by hepatitis is done while the body is trying to detoxify itself of the virus, protecting the liver cell membranes where most of the metabolic activities takes place is crucial. PC inhibits the tendency of stellate cells to progress to cirrhosis. It exhibits anti-fibrotic effects related to the breakdown of collagen. It has been shown to prevent lipid peroxidation associated with liver damage in alcoholic cirrhosis.

Studies show that PC protects the liver against damage from alcoholism, environmental toxins, viruses, and prescription and recreational drugs. Lecithin is found in organ meat, in moderately high amounts in red meats, whole nuts and seeds, soybeans, brewers yeast, fish, wheat germ, legumes, and grains. Dietary supplementation with minimum of about 800 mg daily with meals significantly speeds recovery of the liver. PC is a safe means of supplementing dietary choline.

Choline is a member of the B vitamins group, and prevents the deposition of fats in the liver and facilitates the transport of fats into the cells. Its deficiency leads to degenerative liver diseases like cirrhosis, bleeding, and kidney damage. Cabot (1996) indicated that increases in choline levels in the liver facilitate the synthesis of the enzyme callaginase. Collaginase helps dissolve collagenous scar tissues in cirrhotic patients. In the body, inositol combines with choline to form lecithin. Lecithin increases the levels of choline in the liver, which in turn facilitates the activities of the enzyme collagenase that helps dissolve cirrhotic scar tissues. Dietary sources of choline, which facilitate fat metabolism, are soybeans, nutritional yeast, fish, peanuts, cauliflower, lettuce, cabbage, lentils, chick peas, and brown rice.

What should I do if my doctor wants to put me on statin drugs?
Get your lipid panel and liver enzymes evaluated every three months. During the first three months, follow the following protocol:
- Replace processed foods with organic whole foods.
- Do liver and gall bladder flushes to relieve liver congestions.
- Consume foods rich in fibers, vitamins, and essential fatty acids from apples, bananas, carrots, beans, garlic, brown rice, essential fatty acids, and lots of fibers from fruits, vegetables, soy products, lecithin, raw nuts, oat meals, cereals, and whole grains.
- Reduce free radicals in the liver with antioxidants from green drinks or super food formulas.
- Inculcate herbal and homeopathic remedies that facilitate the movement of bile.
- For cooking, replace vegetable oils with extra virgin ólive, coconut oil, or palm oil.
- Broil and bake instead of frying.
- Do a series of detoxifications through enemas to relieve the work load of the liver.
- Replace margarine, butter, lard, and drippings with low-fat spreads.
- Replace cream and whole milk with organic half-fat versions, organic goat milk, rice milk, soy milk, or skimmed milk.

- Replace creamed cheese with reduced-fat spreads and cottage cheese.
- Replace fatty meats, such as beef, pork, and duck with deep-sea fish, free-range poultry, and organic eggs.
- Replace chips, crisps, and nuts with oven-baked chips.
- Replace biscuits, cakes, and pastries with low-fat alternatives like tea cakes.
- Eat small amounts of low-fat versions of high-fat foods like pizza and lasagna.
- Cook with less fat.
- Skim fat off the surface of soups and casseroles.
- After three months, go and surprise your doctor!

Chapter 3

Living with liver disease

After Your Diagnosis;—What Next?

After being diagnosed with hepatitis, the next step is learning how to live with it instead of dying from it. It is normal to go through the emotional phase of grief after hearing the news that you have an illness you will have to live with the rest of your life. We want you to know that we have been there, and though we don't know how long ago you acquired this virus, you need to know that there is life after liver disease.

"If you help others, you will be helped, perhaps not tomorrow, perhaps in not in one hundred years, but you will be helped. Nature must pay off the debt... it is a mathematical law and all life is mathematics"
Gurdjieff

You can have the best treatment in the world, but if you do not resolve your inner conflicts and replace negative emotional feelings of anger, unforgiving, and blame and with positive mental attitudes, your treatment will only be successful if suppress your symptoms with drugs or if replace your liver through transplantation. Negative emotions will do nothing except block the healing currents that flow restlessly through our thinking. True healing starts with inner peace, acceptance, and understanding. The responsibility for your health rest solely in your hands, and only you know exactly how you feel.

⊠ *Flashback*
Though my wife was told by specialists that I had incurable, progressive-degenerative diseases, she refused to accept the doctor's verdict, refused to be trapped in a cycle of fear of the inevitable, and refused to go through the normal emotional reactions associated with my diagnosis. She focused on my positive prognosis with amazing fortitude. Through her persistent prayers, God transfigured us from the valley of the shadow of death to the hilltop.

The "Why Me" Syndrome

About 45 percent of people living with hepatitis don't know how they were infected. Viruses, as part of God's creations, were created for man; man was not created for the viruses. Like fire, they are good servants and bad masters. Even if you know how you became infected, we want you to know there are no accidents and for every event there is a reason and a positive experience that can be attained. If life gives you hepatitis as a challenge, make it an assignment and use your experience to educate others. Take a clip from a quote by Horace Mann, the first president of Antioch College in Ohio. "Be ashamed to die if you have not won a victory for humanity." Make your experience overcoming hepatitis and liver disease your victory and gift for humanity. You and only you can turn your lemons to lemonade, your weights into wings, and your stumbling blocks into stepping stones. We want you to know that there are no incurable diseases, but there are incurable attitudes. We want you to know that he who fights and runs away lives to fight another day.

⊠ *Flashback*
For us, the only power we had after my diagnosis was the power of perseverance. We decided to make the best of life. We knew there are no gains without pains. We made up our minds to make our experience our assignment to humanity.

The Way Forward

Our illnesses should be a learning experience on how not to be sick again. Our attitudes can handicap and abort our healing. A time of illness is often a time to tap into latent capacities when we turn our thoughts inward and reevaluate our lifestyles. The initial diagnosis is understandably accompanied by fear, but often most of us always have premonitions of what is about to come our way. Anybody can heal if they begin their journey to recovery from the mind-body connection. We know you are at crossroads, and this is a time to take an honest look at the patterns that negate your journey towards recovery. It is time to bid farewell to attitudes, places, or acquaintances that no longer compliment the journey to regain your health. . In her book , *The Wheels of Light,* Rosalyn Bruyere clearly substantiates the above views, "We are no less affected by air pollution, noise pollution, or people pollution...if we are exposed to negative energies for long enough, the potential results will be detrimental to our health—physical, mental, emotional, or spiritual." The decisions we make will either increase or decrease our journey toward health. We want to see you not as an aggregate of organs for the liver specialist to analyze but as a whole person whose emotions are inseparable from his body. "Your current condition is but a cloud that is hiding a shinning sun and as long as you know that the sun is there, there is no reason to get too worked up over the temporary clouds around you." (Myss, 1996).

Getting CURED CONVENTIONALLY Or Getting Healed

Getting cured conventionally or getting healed of a disease is another decision we have to make to be able to move forward. We are going to come across remedies and doctors that relieve us of our physical pains. Often times, this is a passive process that occurs without our participation. We yield to the attending physical authority who offers any remedy that will alleviate our predicaments. Often times, when we approach our illness with this approach, drugs and surgery do all the work. In her book, anatomy of the spirit, Caroline Myss (1996) points out that when a person is passive with an attitude of "just do it for me", he does not fully heal; he may recover, but he may never deal fully with the source of his illnesses. On the other hand, an active participation on our part in our health care means we understand our body, the disease, and the reasons for any therapeutic regimen by the attending physician. True healing emphasizes our attitudes over our aptitudes as our attitudes influence our affluence. It goes beyond being a spectator to the disease to being actively involved in healing our attitudes and correcting our negative patterns internally to repair our emotional injuries. When we consciously turn our attention from our illness and contemplate wellness, something begins to happen in the realm of the mind and spirit that reinforces our desire to overcome our adversities. Gradually, we realize, as Dr. Frederic Bailes puts it, *"There is a power in man that can lift him toward his highest aspirations and make him the person he wants to be. No enslavement can hold a person, no illness can defeat him, when he comes to understand the tremendous power that lies within him just waiting to be released."*

You have to come to a point where you want to manage your health and not the disease so that transplantation will be the last resort and not the first option. We believe if you change your nutritional status, your thought patterns, and your life styles, you can stop the progression of liver disease. Since life is about choices, the choices you make now will determine the life you will live tomorrow. We want to encourage you to tap into the regenerative capacities of the liver and make the best of what is left if you have de-compensated cirrhosis. *The liver can still carry on its normal functions even if 75 percent of its tissue has been permanently damaged(Palmer, 2004).*

Maximizing Your Support System
- Discuss your diagnosis with your spouse, partner, or immediate family members. You need all the support you can get.
- Retrace your steps: Try to identify how you got infected, fill in the gaps, and tidy loose ends.
- Protect people you come in contact with daily with vaccinations. You need them to be healthy enough to support you.
- Wash your hands with soap after touching your own blood or body fluids like tissues, menstrual pads, tampons, or bandages. Clean all blood spills with bleach.
- All sores and open sores should be covered with bandages.
- Wear gloves and use bleach to properly clean any area that your blood and/or body fluids have been exposed to.
- Make positive changes to your life. Re-evaluate past or current behaviors that predisposed you to the illness.
- Become an informed patient. In becoming an informed patient, use the Internet and yellow pages as your primary source of information for local health food stores and alternative doctors in your area.
- Buy books on hepatitis B on the Internet or at health food stores.
- Do not use herbs without consulting with a primary-care provider or a holistic practitioner.
- If you are pregnant, tell your doctor you have liver disease or hepatitis.
- Monitor the state of your liver, check for liver cirrhosis, and/or cancer every six months.
- Have periodic alpha-fetoprotein blood tests and an ultrasound for liver cancer.
- Stay away from Tylenol.

How Do I Find A Liver Specialist?
Most likely, your first contact with a liver specialist might be a referral from your primary care doctor, from the emergency room if you rush in for unexplained illness, when donating blood, by word of mouth, or from

a referral list from your insurance company. Even if you do not have much control over your choice of doctors, you still can ask questions.

"A good doctor is one who is open, curious, passionate and most importantly not afraid to learn"
William Finley Green., A hepatitis B survivor

- You liver doctor will either be a gastroenterologist or a hepatologist and infectious diseases specialist. (A gastroenterologist is an internist who specializes in digestive diseases; a hepatologist is a medical doctor who has taken special training programs that emphasize liver diseases. There is currently no board certifying examination to become a hepatologist; an infectious disease specialist is an internist who specializes in treating infectious diseases.)

- Your progress involve having an open, trust-based relationship with your doctor. Good communication is a two-way street that is mutually beneficial to you and your doctor.

- Watch for experience, flexibility, open mindedness, and personality in your doctor. She must be one who will be patient with you before making you a patient. It will benefit you if your doctor put himself or herself in your position and understands how you feel.

- You do not have to be an observer in you health care; you can be an active participant.

- You do not want doctors who only talk *to* you, but who will not talk with you.

- You want to clearly understand where you are, physically, and how liver disease interacts with, relates to, and affects other health conditions you have and the medications you take.

- You need to ask your doctor about the anticipated outcomes of the specific medications you are prescribed, in addition to your own use of Internet research on the indications and adverse reactions of the medications. More detailed information on your medications can also be obtained from your pharmacist.

- You want to know your viral load, liver enzyme levels, stage of your liver damage, your prognosis, adverse reactions of drugs, risks and benefits of drugs, and procedures that will be followed. Ask questions about new drugs and experimental procedures, and evaluate their necessity. Strand (2003) strongly recommends that patients not take any drug that has not been on the market for a minimum of five years.

- Document your progress as you receive treatment. Note adverse reactions to medications and discuss you feelings about your findings with your doctor.
- You want to know your doctor's opinion about alternative remedies and the role of nutrition in chronic degenerative liver diseases.
- With this book and other similar books written by qualified medical personnel on hepatitis and liver diseases, discuss with your doctor if you will be allowed to discus adjunct therapies and possible herb-drug interactions.
- If your doctor is not knowledgeable about alternative therapies, ask if s (he) would be willing to co-manage your conditions with a holistic practitioner. If not, show the doctor your independent research. If the doctor is still uninterested, look for a holistic-friendly doctor. Please see the resources listed below.
- Always update your primary healthcare provider with information about your treatments with your liver doctor.
- Herbs do interact with some conventional medicines, especially interferon. Your doctor needs to be involved in your decision to use alternative therapies to let you know if it is working or if it is time to try other options.
- Take a clue from the experience of author Norman Cousins, as described in his book, *Anatomy of an Illness*. He counted himself lucky to be associated with a doctor who recognized that his most important obligation to his patient was to encourage to the fullest the patient's will to live, and to mobilize the natural resources of the body and mind to overcome his otherwise incurable disease. Cousins' doctor believed that active involvement was key to recovery. His doctor was open to the wide varieties of alternatives proposed.
- "If you get the distinct impression that your doctor is annoyed with you, makes you feel like you are a bother, doesn't know how to treat your illness properly, and covers that up by making you feel stupid, refuses to listen to new information that you try to share, won't let you get a second opinion without feeling

threatened, then you need a new doctor because your doctor should work for you" (Green, 2002)

Resources to locate holistic practitioners
- Healing Centers United: www.healingcentersunited.org
- American Holistic Medical Association: www.holisticmedicine.org
- Holistic Health Network :www.holisticnetwork.org
- To find a naturopathic doctor: www.heartspring.net
- American Holistic Health Association: www.ahha.org
- Alternative health professionals: www.healthprofs.com

What I Need To Know Before Choosing A Holistic Practitioner:
- Before deciding to use an alternative therapy, determine what your expectations are and why conventional medicine has not fulfilled you expectations.
- Independently research how the remedy works and the potential risks and benefits associated with your treatment.

  "I refuse to accept the idea that man is mere flotsams and jetsam in the river of life unable to influence the unfolding events which surround him"
  Martin Luther King Jr.

- Since the majority of alternative therapies are not covered by insurance, check with your insurance carrier to see what treatments are covered. Some insurance carriers offer discounts for acupuncture, chiropractic care, and massage therapy. It is best to seek holistic practitioners who accept your insurance.
- Locate and interview holistic practitioners as you would your liver specialist.
- Because most of your services may not be covered by mainstay insurance, work with holistic practitioners who can guide you in choosing the best herbal remedy for your illness, while taking you stomach tolerance and budget into consideration.

Online resources for finding doctors
- www.findadoc.com is a resource for information about doctors' training and certifications.

- www.healthgrades.com is a resource for malpractice judgments and licensing board actions.
- www.abms.org is the Internet resource of the American Board of Medical Specialties (ABMS) and a resource for information about doctors' board certifications. Their phone number is (866) 275-2267.
- Another resource for malpractice judgments, sanctions, and disciplinary actions, by state licensing boards, is the American Medical Association link

www.ama-assn/ama/pub/category/2645.html. It has direct links to all state boards.

- For cancer terminology and treatment options, visit www.caring4cancer.com.
- For information on commonly-used drugs, visit www.rxlist.com.
- Others: www.centerwatch.com; www.epocrates.com; www.drugs.com; and www.lexi.com

How Do I Predict Adverse Reactions Of Prescription Drugs?

I strongly recommend asking your doctor about genetic testing to see if you have reactions to any prescribed medications. This will help you map predictable paths, reveal occult adverse reactions, and possibly save your life.

Before filling drug prescriptions, a simple life-saving gene analysis test can be done to reduce adverse reactions associated with conventional drugs and to check their compatibility with your system. In a 2005 number of *Vital Health News Journal*, Dr. Allen Roses, worldwide vice-president of genetics at GlaxoSmithKline (GSK) said, "Some of the most expensive drugs work on fewer than half of the patients for which they are prescribed. This is due to genetics interfering in some way with the medicine." He proposes a future industry in which a patient will undergo a simple and cheap genetic test that determines whether or not the patient will benefit from a particular drug. He thinks this approach will never be implemented because it goes against a marketing culture within the drug industry of "selling as many drugs as possible to the greatest number of patients." (Reese, 2005) Dr. Bob Water buttressed these views in the May 2004 issue of *Readers' Digest* when he indicated that the absence of genetic testing is costing Americans an estimated 100,000 deaths annually. This makes prescription medications the sixth leading cause of death in America.

Doctors Health advisory: Because liver disease follows a very unpredictable path, changes do take place over a short period of time, so it is advisable to get a second opinion about your treatment modalities because misdiagnosis occurs. Shopping around for opinions from different specialist or web-based doctors is counterproductive. Neglecting the underlying condition while looking for a doctor to tell you what you want to hear might compromise your health. One should be able to make a decision based on the professional opinions of two to three specialists.

The Grim Statistics

- The famous Indian doctor Shevananda was quoted as saying that 99 percent of all health disorders and degenerative diseases are attributable to dysfunctional liver.
- In 1961, there were 72,000 documented case of hepatitis, making it the highest incidence for any year since the disease had first begun to be reported in 1952.
- The American Liver Foundation (ALF) estimates that liver disease affects one in every ten Americans. This amounts to about 30 million Americans.
- One in 100,000 people has a truly healthy liver in the United States. (Tipps, 2002)
- Liver disease is the fourth leading cause of death in America. (Hobbs, 2002)
- Currently, 25,000 Americans die each year of liver cirrhosis, a complication of progressive liver disease, making it the seventh leading cause of death in America.
- Predictions suggest that there will be a 60 percent increase in the incidence of liver cirrhosis, a 68 percent increase in the incidence of liver cancer, a 528 percent increase in the need for transplantation, and a 223 percent increase in liver death rate in the United States.

The aim of this book is to slow or stop the progression of the disease and change the medical mind set from a "cut-it–out" mentality and a drug-prescription ritual to non-toxic and non-invasive approaches, i.e. an ounce of prevention is better than a pound of cure approach.

Chapter 4

Managing complications of liver disease

Managing Acute and Chronic Symptoms Of Liver Disease
Acute symptoms

The symptoms of acute hepatitis infection include vomiting, nausea, loss of appetite, fatigue, and jaundice. These symptoms are manifested because of temporary disruption of the daily activities of the liver

"Acidosis, predicated by malnutrition, is the etiology of all degenerative diseases"
Bob Barefoot (2002)

cells. Joint and abdominal pains may accompany an acute infection. In acute hepatitis, the immune system eradicates the virus from the body. Tests will manifest the presence of hepatitis antibodies in the blood, indicating previous attacks. During acute hepatitis infection, extra nutrition is needed to prevent unplanned weight loss. This may include more calories and a protein diet. Protein drinks and shakes are advisable at this time.

Liver Cirrhosis and Chronic symptoms

Depression. Because of the inability of the liver to clear toxins from the blood, accumulation of ammonia in the brain leads to mental disturbances, memory loss, malaise, and depression.

Fibrosis occurs when injuries to the liver cells start affecting the protective covering (collagen) encompassing and in between the liver cells. This is referred to as bridging. As the collagenous tissues become thicker and harder than normal liver tissues, it becomes fibrotic and nodular (lumpy). This fibrotic tissue is referred to as scar. These scar tissues are dead tissues. As the inflammation and irritation continues, there is more scar formation as dead liver cells harden into non-functioning scar tissues (fibrosis) that replaces normal healthy liver cells.

Healthy liver cells do not have many stellate cells, so they do not have as much scar tissues as inflamed cells. The liver cells called stellate cells produce the scar tissue which protects against ongoing inflammation. The liver can still function as the remaining healthy liver cells often take over the activities of the dead cells. As this process continues, new liver cells try to grow from the injured cells but are prevented by the scar or fibrotic tissues.

Cirrhosis is derived from the Greek word meaning "tawny" or "orange." It was first introduced by an individual called Laennec in 1826. He used it to classify a condition where the functional size of the liver is reduced to about one third of it's usual size and with its outer surface covered by a series of fawn-colored small grains of varying sizes, from that of a millet seed to that of a hemp seed, and having a soft leather sensation to touch. (Greene, 2002)

Injuries from the attacking virus, overzealous inflammatory responses from the immune system, and toxins lead to the formation of nodules in the liver combine with fibrous tissues to alter the liver's architecture. Extensive fibrosis progresses to cirrhosis. The functions of the liver in cirrhosis are further hampered as attempts at regeneration takes place. If the fibrotic tissues extend far enough to alter the function and integrity of the liver, physical manifestations of the disease set in. The extensive scars constrict the liver tissues, reducing its structure, functionality, and usable size. Blood and lymph can no longer transverse the liver. At this stage the liver is said to be cirrhotic.

In the early stage of liver cirrhosis, the liver is not damaged by the complications. This early stage is called compensated cirrhosis i.e. compensatory mechanisms are developed by the body to enable the liver to continue to function under these dire circumstances. Individuals with compensated cirrhosis exhibit little or no symptoms, and nutrient needs are similar to those with hepatitis infection or pre-cirrhosis.

☒ *Flashback*
I had an accumulation of fluids in my abdomen (ascites) and in my legs and hands (peripheral edema.)

How do I know if I have extensive scarring?

- elevated iron levels, especially in individual with chronic hepatitis C
- elevated alpha fetoprotein
- low platelet count
- prolonged prothrombin time
- elevated liver enzymes
- positive clinical finding on biopsy
- all acute symptoms of hepatitis
- reduction in bile duct secretion interferes with fat metabolism
- reduction in carbohydrate metabolism exacerbates diabetes
- reduction in lipoproteins metabolism; lower blood cholesterol

As chronic hepatitis progresses, patients may experience loss of appetite, increasing fatigue and reduction in physical activity because the liver is unable to manufacture essential proteins or converts carbohydrates to usable energy. Despite increased nutritional needs, eating becomes a challenge. When complications progress to liver failure, we have de-compensated cirrhosis. At this stage, the ability of the liver to compensate for the ongoing damage is gone. If cirrhosis is caught in the early stages, when scarring is minimal, appropriate treatment applied, and individuals make the required lifestyles change, cirrhosis can be reversed. Reversing cirrhosis becomes almost impossible when there is decomposition (Palmer, 2004). Studies show that if 75% of a healthy liver removed, the remaining portion of the liver will expand to occupy the empty space until the initial weight is attained. The liver will then return to its original functional capacity. Alternatively, if the remaining portion is permanently damaged or scarred as in decompensated cirrhosis, regeneration would not take place.

Norman Cousins (1979) sees scar formation as a natural recuperative mechanism of the body as it responds to injury. Whenever we get injured, nature protects us with scar formation as a repair mechanism. It is like putting a patch on your flat tire. It is nature's normal response to protect its creation. Cousins sees the normal response of scar formation as the body's response that aims to restore normalcy, produce lasting immunity, and sees its outcome as a lasting chance to make the organism better prepared to face future challenges. "He indicated that the scarred part of the body was better able to resist the insult that caused scarring." (Cousins, p. 16). In chronic hepatitis, we have an overzealous immunological response that is not commensurate with the injury. In this case, when we have multiple patches on our tire, we see a reduction in the functional ability of the tire, and the repair shop recommends outright replacement which translates to liver transplantation.

⊠ *Flashback*
Luckily my situation was an exception to medical norms. I had de-compensated cirrhosis, and I am doing excellent. A liver disease protocol without detoxification and metabolic waste management regimen is like a cat without claws.

Cirrhotic patients can manifest liver palms (palmar erythema), characterized by bright red coloring of the palms, enlarged blood vessels in the upper chest, back, face, and arms, that look like little red spiders, known as spider angiomatas. Women may have reduced under-arm hair; men may have breast enlargement. Terry's nails—completely white brittle nails—may occur.

⊠ *Flashback*
My nails became very brittle and white, which is a classic symptom of progressive liver disease. The implication of this is that I was in a chronic state of liver failure. I could not excrete bilirubin through the bile ducts. Consequently, I could not metabolize fat and oils, was completely jaundiced, and my skin was yellow like mustard. The circulating bilirubin throughout my body caused yellowing of my skin, urine, and the white part of the eye. I began to loose proteins, coupled with ammonia toxicity. My weight dropped to 109 pounds in February of 2004. I could not get up from the bed, and I had to use the bedpan to relieve myself. By this time, my doctors determined that I was totally disabled, and it was assumed that I would be incapacitated for the rest of my life. I could not compensate for these changes, and I was recommended for total disability. I developed spontaneous bacterial peritonitis several times, which required hospitalization in the I.C.U. and emergency intravenous (IV) antibiotics.

Meeting nutritional needs of patients with decompensated cirrhosis
Common nutrition problems associated with de-compensated cirrhosis are malnutrition, indigestion, inadequate intake of nutrients, and mal-

absorption. These are best managed with frequent meals of with small-portion, dense, high-energy and high-protein diets. Frequent food intake may be helpful in trying to maximize the dietary intake of individuals with cirrhosis. Foods can be fortified with other energy dense and/or protein-dense ingredients to increase energy and protein intake without increasing food volume. Oral protein energy supplements may be helpful as adjunct to regular diets. Low-iron multivitamin and mineral supplement are recommended when food intake is inadequate.

Doctors Health Advisory: Individual with de-compensated cirrhosis should abstain from red meat altogether and explore vegetarian diets.
- 60 percent of the diet should be from complex carbohydrates to supply energy needs
- 30 percent of proteins should be from vegetable sources and lean meat (fish and poultry)
- Eight to ten 8-ounce glasses of water daily
- 1000 – 1500 mg of sodium daily
- Twenty percent of essential fatty acids daily
- Lots of organic fruits and vegetables

Portal Hypertension

If cirrhosis progresses to the point where very few functional cells are left, the extensive scarring makes it impossible for fluids to pass through the liver, and metabolic abilities of the liver are hampered. Pressure back up is created in the portal vein. This condition is known as portal hypertension. A cirrhotic liver is like a mangled soda can. The liver often tries to regenerate from this condition, leaving abnormal architectural patterns, which is like trying to straighten out the mangled soda can. Internally, shunt vessels are developed in the esophagus which bleed easily. In the tiny blood vessels in the sinusoids where metabolic exchange between the liver cells occurs, nutrients and toxins are disrupted, and circulation is gradually cut off. Back-flow pressure is generated if blood entering the liver cannot pass through. Portal venous pressure increases and ultimately exceeds systemic venous pressure. Metabolic activities are hampered, the liver is further undermined, and nutrients are not supplied to the liver. This build up of pressure is transferred to neighboring vessels which causes dilation of the vessels in the spleen, stomach, esophagus, and extremities. Gastric and esophageal varices are not designed to handle the pressure of this extra flow, so they rupture easily, causing internal bleeding and bleeding in the mouth. Fluids leak and accumulate in the abdomen. This is referred to as *ascites*.

Ascites predisposes individuals to infection as toxic fluids hang around the body longer. Infections associated with these fluids are referred to as bacteria peritonitis. If the ascites is associated with fever and stomach pains, spontaneous bacterial peritonitis is suspected. This occurs when bacteria in the colon infects fluids in the stomach. There may be protrusion of the belly button which can burst due to leakage of ascitic fluid. This condition is called umbilical hernia. This also leads to rupture and bleeding in the veins of the esophagus and stomach. Esophageal and gastric varices occur, with increased pressure in portal circulation. Blood flows backward from portal circulation into the systemic venous circulatory system where they are connected at certain points. Some of these connections occur in the stomach and the esophagus. This leads to varicose veins in the stomach and the esophagus, hemorrhoids in the rectum, and under the skin on the abdomen known as caput medusa, during which dilated blood vessels can come out of the belly button. Back up pressures in the portal veins hamper the passage of nutrients to the liver and the metabolism of bile. This ultimately hampers the supply of nutrients to the liver and the synthesis of fat-soluble vitamins. This is managed with intravenous fluids and blood transfusions. A domino effect causes serious symptoms and deficiencies through the body that include jaundice caused by the inability of the liver to excrete bilirubin, the yellowish bile pigment. This cause yellowing of the skin, urine, and the white of the eye. This causes high bilirubin levels of more than 2mg/dL.

⊠ *Flashback*
I had developed varices in the esophagus which burst quite often, leading to profuse and uncontrollable vomiting of blood. This condition referred to as hematemesis was a life-threatening condition that required my hospitalization. Studies show that about 30 percent of episodes of hematemesis results in death. Glad to be here!

Why do liver patients itch?
Inflammatory liver disease is associated with the inability of the liver to eliminate toxins from the body. This often leads to accumulation of normal substances like endogenous opoids, known as enkaphalins, found in the blood plasma, which causes pruritis (itching) in liver-disease patients.

Cryoglobulinemia occur when the cirrhotic liver produces defective proteins, which can damage the nervous system and the kidneys and cause persistent itching. This is conventionally managed with antihistamines.

How do I manage salt intake with my liver disease?
The inability of the liver to synthesis albumin from amino acids hampers the function of this important protein that regulates fluids levels in the body. This ultimately leads to fluids leaking out of the vessels into the legs, abdomen, and other extremities, causing fluid retention. Fluid retention is caused by the inability of the liver to manufacture the protein albumin that regulates fluid balance. Cirrhosis disturbs the regulation of body sodium and water balance, and excessive retention of sodium drives accumulation of fluids. When this occurs in the legs it is referred to as *edema*. Infections of the fluids are referred to as spontaneous bacterial *peritonitis*. Salt disrupts the functional ability of cirrhotic livers to regulate fluid balance by making the liver send inappropriate hormonal signals which disrupt the salt water balance of the body. Salt absorbs water like a sponge, thus retaining fluids in the body .This ultimately leads to edema and ascites. Conversely, potassium help dispel fluids from the body.

Low-salt diet and diuretics like spironlactone (Aldactone™) and furosemide (Lasix™) are employed to manage fluid retentions. Sodium is needed to help sustain fluid balance in the body, and is supplied from foods and vegetables. Commercially-available table salt is called sodium chloride. Sodium chloride is a devitalized product that is often enriched with iodine. I do not recommend this product for human consumption. The standard American diet supplies about 35 times the RDA of salt derived from table salt, curried meats, canned foods, and outdoor dining. The food processing industry is doing a great injustice to Americans with the way foods are processed with sodium. One of the reasons for increased blood pressure is the over-consumption of salt and under-consumption of potassium-rich foods that maintain the sodium – potassium balance needed to maintain normal blood pressure in arteries. This shift in osmotic balance is responsible for hypertension.

In their book about how to prevent and treat cancer with natural medicine, Drs. Michael Murray, Tim Birdcall, Joseph Pizzorno, and Paul Riley (2002) indicate that a disproportionate consumption of sodium over potassium and other essential nutrients creates imbalances in the body that increases our susceptibility to cancer. Individuals with liver cirrhosis and ascites are often put on salt restriction. It this case, sea salt or rock salt are better options because they are unrefined and natural. Sea salt is naturally evaporated, is richer in flavor and minerals, and adheres better to food than refined table salt. Because of these characteristics, you need less of sea salt to get the same flavor. Nutritionists believe that for every gram of sodium consumed, about 220 mL of fluids are retained by the body. Hence, lower consumption of salt results in lower fluid retention. *Individual with advanced liver disease and ascites need to the restricted to between 500 – 1500 mg of salt per day. One spoon of table salt contains about 2,300 mg of sodium.*

Synthetic diuretics like lasix are used to increase urine flow and to reduce fluid retention in cases of de-compensated cirrhosis, which also adversely reduces the body's potassium level. This has to be restored using potassium supplements. Under professional supervision, alternative-care practitioners use whole dandelion leaves, which are potent diuretics that contain potassium, to synergistically replace that which is lost—a classical case of synergy.

Individuals with ascites and de-compensated cirrhosis should avoid the following foods:
- food from fast-food stores
- food from Chinese restaurants
- canned foods
- foods with high-salt contents listed on their labels
- processed foods
- curried meats
- red meats
- salt substitutes containing potassium chloride

Cooking for liver disease patients
- use sea salt or rock salt sparingly
- use spices and food seasonings instead of salt
- Cook with small amounts of sea salt, rock salt, or salt alternatives available in grocery stores.
- Do not to add salt to prepared foods.
- Use stock cubes, bouillon cubes, or gravy granules in cooking in lieu of salt
- Avoid packaged or canned soups, if possible.
- Replace canned vegetables with frozen vegetables.

- Avoid cured meats, including ham, bacon, sausages, and salami.
- Use cooked fresh free-range meat, poultry, or eggs.
- Avoid pre-pared meals and sauces that are high in salt.

If diuretics do not relieve ascites, the abdominal swelling becomes painful and patients have difficulties breathing due to compression on the diaphragm. Paracentesis is indicated. This procedure involves draining fluids from the abdomen through a process called parasynthesis.

⊠ *Flashback*

My stomach had distended to the point that I had umbilical and double ingual hernias. I could neither stand nor walk. I had to undergo umbilical and hiatal-hernia surgery, which left me with permanent post-operative pains in my groin area. My doctor agreed to do the surgery after consultations with ten surgeons within and outside the hospital health system. My health and physical condition made me a high-risk patient for any form of such an invasive procedure. A one-inch incision was made on my abdomen to rearrange my impacted colon. The cirrhotic and fibro tic scars that formed on my liver were likened to what an alcoholic would acquire over a period of 15 years or a drug addict over 10 years.

Hepatic encephalopathy

When liver cells are damaged by disease, the liver's role is of the liver in the conversion of amino acids into proteins is compromised. Proteins are the building blocks that the liver utilizes to manufacture all of the body components and the important part of the immune system called the antibodies that help overwhelm infective agents. Proteins also serve as alternative energy sources under dire situations such as when the body is breaking down its own muscles, desperate to stay alive. When the amount of proteins intake exceeds the liver's ability to process them, there is a build up of nitrogenous wastes, such as ammonia.

A cirrhotic liver cannot convert the by products of protein metabolism, like ammonia, into urea. Ammonia builds up in the body, poisons the brain, and causes mental changes like confusion and, in extreme cases, comas. This condition is referred to as hepatic encephalopathy or impaired mental function. Hepatic encephalopathy is thought to be caused by the build up of protein breakdown products, which the impaired liver has trouble processing. Drug treatment for hepatic encephalopathy is with lactulose, a sugar that is not absorbed from the intestine. It acts as a laxative. It increases dietary protein tolerance by promoting defecation. It expels nitrogen-containing compounds from the gut before bacteria can metabolize them into toxic substances that the liver cannot clear from the system. Lactulose also makes the inside of the gut less acidic, making it impossible for nitrogen-containing toxins and ammonia to be absorbed. An antibiotic, neomycin, may be employed to kill bacteria in the gut. Normal ammonia level should be less than 50 mg/dL. Normal white blood levels are 6,000+, hematocrit 40+, and platelets 150,000+.

⊠ *Flashback*
I had been put on lactulose to clear the excess ammonia that was making me act confused, lasix and adaltone to help me get rid of excess water in my body, Epivir to reduce my viral load, and Prevacid for appetite control. These were al forl palliative care.

Meeting nutritional needs of encephalopathy patients
Dietary modifications for hepatic encephalopathy patients include
- a low-protein diet obtained primarily from plant sources;
- frequent small meals, four to seven times per day, including evening snacks, to enhance nitrogen balance;
- avoiding consumption of large amounts of protein at one meal; and
- Filling up with minimally-processed starch foods and complex carbohydrates for energy or high-calorie drinks.

Why do cirrhotic patients experience fatigue?
Fatigue experienced by individuals with liver disease occurs when an already distressed liver is not getting enough complex carbohydrates for energy, and has to use extra effort to convert food to energy from other sources, like proteins and fats. To keep energy constant during the day, nutritionists recommend small meals consisting of about 60 percent complex carbohydrates which ensure a steady supply of carbohydrates for fuel and energy. This contrasts with simple carbohydrates which are quickly converted into glucose. Glucose reacts chemically with proteins and destroy their ability to function, according to Allan and Lutz (2000). With simple carbohydrates, you get a quick high and a sharp low and the body starts scrambling again for energy from other sources.

Why do cirrhotic patient bleed easily?

The tendency to bleed occurs when the cirrhotic liver cannot manufacture specialized proteins like blood-clotting factors. The prothrombin time, the time needed for the blood to coagulate, is increased. This makes individuals bleed easily, and the bleeding takes longer to stop. This also causes the smaller vessels in the stomach, esophagus, and large intestine to bleed more easily. Similarly, when individuals engage in normal activities like shaving or get other minor irritations, they bleed more easily.

The back flow of blood into the spleen leads to the trapping of platelets, making the platelet count fall. Vitamin K is often administered to help with the production of clotting factors. Fresh frozen plasma containing clotting factors and other proteins is also used. Platelet transfusions are often given to patients with low platelet counts. Infections occur in people with cirrhosis due to depressed immunity to diseases.

Malnutrition, loss of appetite, and weight loss are common with people with progressive cirrhosis. They cannot manufacture fat-soluble vitamins. This causes nausea when foods with fats are eaten. Stored fats cannot be broken down, and streaks of stored fats are visible on the liver causing a condition called fatty liver. Fat may also be excreted in the stool, which is visible as white bands called *steatorrhe*.

Individuals with damaged livers often have thyroid problems since the liver controls the levels of the thyroid hormones. *Cachexia* occurs in individuals with cirrhosis. They generally have loss of muscle mass. This is noticeable in the temporal muscles on the sides of the head, just in front of the ear lobes. In men, breast enlargement (gynecomastia) occurs because of a disruption in the manufacture of estrogen. Impotence and atrophy of the testes occurs because the damaged liver cannot metabolize estrogens. There is lower libido and sexual dysfunction. Metabolism of triglycerides, cholesterol, and sugar are impaired, and various complications from the deficiencies of these nutrients occur.

Doctors Health advisory: Cirrhotic patient's who use blood thinners, aspirin, and non-steroidal anti-inflammatory drugs should be under strict medical supervision due to bleeding propensities.

How I kept liver cancer at bay?

Unless there is a lifestyle change, including abstinence from illicit drug use, red meats, stress, standard American diets, and alcohol, cirrhotic patients gradually progress to *hepatocellular carcinoma*. In advanced cirrhosis, known as end-stage liver cirrhosis, liver transplantation is the only remedy.

Cancer is a degenerative disease caused by a multitude of factors that influence the environment inside the body. Nutrition alone is just a half measure in dealing with cancer. It is the interplay of genetics, stagnation, stress, emotions, and food that has to be addressed in order to provide an environment for healing to take place, instead of only curing the symptoms. The most important part of the immune system is the lymphatic system. Nutrients, herbs, and exercise that facilitate lymphatic flow are critical to relieving the liver of toxins and facilitating its repair.

Though de-compensated cirrhosis is thought to be non-reversible, the progression to cancer can be stopped or drastically slowed if individuals modify their lifestyles. I knew that for me to keep cancer at bay, I had to

"Cancer cells demonstrate a 3 to 5 fold increase in glucose uptake compared to healthy cells" (Demetrakopoulos)

- do bi-weekly coffee or herbal retention enemas or quarterly colonics,
- eliminate red meat from my diet,
- consume only free-range organic chicken and wild-caught sea foods,
- replace table salt with rock salt or sea salt,
- replace white sugar with raw honey or raw brown sugar used sparingly,
- replace white bread with whole wheat bread or sourdough bread,
- stop taking alcoholic beverages,
- never use tobacco,
- stay away from non-prescription drugs,
- stay away from tap water,
- replace cow's milk with goat milk, rice milk and soy milk,
- stay away from carbonated drinks,
- drink organic juices,
- use fortified powdered green foods,

- avoid preservatives and pesticide-grown foods,
- take milk thistle, selenium, medicinal mushrooms and olive leaf extract daily,
- drank 6 – 8 glasses of purified water daily,
- reduce my risk to environmental, household and occupational toxins,
- avoid other of risk factors,
- maintain excellent digestive health,
- replace hydrogenated oils, vegetable oils and trans fatty acids with organic cold-pressed extra virgin olive oil and coconut oil,
- consume substantial amounts of essential fatty acids,
- stay away from fast foods and fried foods,
- exercise regularly to reduce the glucose (sugar) demands of cancer cells, and
- Do cheat occasionally on all of the above.

From the writings of two-time winner of the Nobel Prize in Medicine, Otto Warburg, I found that cancer cells love sugar and acidic environments and hate oxygen and sunlight. I used raw honey sparingly, did at least ten deep outdoor breathing exercises daily, and used Hoxley and Essiac anti-cancer herbal formulas. I succeeded in creating alkaline internal environments that defy infective pathogens and cancer cells. The hepatitis viruses inhabit the liver, and the bold antibodies that fight them are derived from the lymphatic system. By restoring liver strength and cleaning the blood and lymphatic system with blood and lymphatic tonic, I reduce my viral loads and prevented the progression of cirrhotic changes.

Primary benign tumors or cysts are seen frequently and differential diagnosis is done to rule out cancer. Primary liver cancers are mostly caused by a fungus or chronic hepatitis that has progressed to cirrhosis.

Studies indicate that it takes an average of 30 years from the date of initial infection and about 10 years after the development of cirrhosis for the development of liver cancer. Individuals with liver cirrhosis have a 20 percent probability of developing liver cancer within 10 years of developing cirrhosis.

Like pulling a plant from the soil and leaving it out in fresh air and sunlight to wither and dehydrate so too do cancer cells suffer when we deprive them of sugar. They also shrink from oxygen and sunlight like roaches shrinking from daylight.

⊠ *Flashback*

When I was diagnosed with diffuse large-cell non-Hodgkin's lymphoma, I thought the "Big C" meant a death sentence. Cancer of the lymph nodes is one of the most aggressive lymphomas with malignant tendencies. Many people with lymphoma have no symptoms until it has advanced to its late stages and is inoperable and unresponsive to treatment. It can be spread through the lymph nodes to other organs. Lymphoma typically metastasizes to the liver, the brain, and the bones where symptoms appear as headaches, seizures, vomiting, and liver pain. The difficulty of and delay in diagnosing lymphoma, the ambiguity of the symptoms, and the lack of early detection means that, for many people, a diagnosis is a death sentence. Sadly, few advances in lymphoma cancer treatment have been made even though it kills more people annually than most other cancers combined. Non-Hodgkin's lymphoma (NHL) is the most common cancer of the lymphatic system, according to the Lymphoma Research Foundation. The environmental health perspective indicates that increases in NHL incidences are linked to the presence of environmental toxins, solvents, shampoos, pesticides, and insecticides like DDT, PCB, and a whole variety of home and occupational toxins that find their way into the human body. Since the early 1970s, the incidence of NHL has nearly doubled, and between 1973 and 1998, new cases of NHL seen each year escalated almost 83 percent. The American Cancer Foundation estimates that in 2006, approximately 58,000 new cases of NHL were diagnosed, and 18,840 Americans died from the disease. NHL starts from the lymph nodes or a specialized lymph organ such as the spleen. Since lymphocytes can circulate to all parts of the body through the lymph vessels and blood stream, abnormal lymphocyte can reach any part of the body. For me, chemotherapy and radiation treatments are like resolving a domestic dispute with nuclear weapons. The months of chemotherapy turned out to be the greatest pain in my life and a tremendous family burden.

The American Liver Foundation states that end-stage liver diseases, such as liver cancer, more than doubled between 1979 and 1998, and the number is expected to double again over the next 10 – 20 years. Metastatic liver cancer occurs when a primary cancer has progressed to other areas. Similarly, cancers that originate primarily from the lungs, digestive tract, and the breast areas can metastasize to the liver. We believe that *cancer is cancer* whether it originates from the liver or elsewhere in the body. All humans produce cancer cells. Cancer develops when the rate of production is higher than the rate of the destruction of those cells. They grow where there is long-standing malnutrition, psychosomatic stress, internal pollution, dehydration, sedentary lifestyle, and hypoxia or lack of oxygen.

The American Association for the Study of Liver Disease (AASLD) recommends screening for hepatic tumors every six months when chronic hepatitis infection are present in men older than 45 years old, in patients with biopsy-proven cirrhosis, and in patients with a family history of liver cancer.

End-stage cirrhosis is an indication for liver transplantation. Rejection occurs when the individual's immune system sees the donor liver as foreign. Transplanted livers are not bio-synergistically compatible with the host's livers. This can cause the donor liver to be destroyed. All transplant patients are *"Inadequate exposure to sunlight is an important risk factor in the development and metastasis of cancer especially in the western hemisphere" Flora A. bade.* required to take immunosuppressive drugs and steroids like prednisone and azathioprine, which suppress an already-compromised immune system. About 10 percent of patients who undergo transplantation develop chronic rejection that does not respond to drugs. A second transplantation is the only available option. Because the immune system is suppressed with drugs, infections are very common in transplanted patients. Autoimmune hepatitis and primary biliary cirrhosis generally recur in the new liver. Patients with cirrhosis from hepatitis B or C are at risk for the new liver to become infected with the virus. There is a relatively high probability of new livers developing cirrhosis if the factors that caused hepatitis and inflammations are not addressed from a nutritional and mental health point of view. Hepatocellular carcinoma is similarly caused by mycotoxins (aflatoxins), a metabolite of fungus. aspergillus that contaminates foods, such as peanuts, grains, and beans. It is very common in Africa and Asia. Individuals with liver disease will need to have a blood test for liver cancer and an ultrasound of the liver every six months.

How do I screen for liver cancer?

Alpha-fetoprotein This fetoprotein is a protein that regenerative cancer or liver cells secrete into the blood. Increased blood levels of this protein are a signal for lurking liver cancer. High alpha-fetoprotein, above 500 ng/mL, and sustained rise of this protein on serial measurements is suspicious and confirmed with radiologic tests like a CT scan, angiography, or MRI.

☒ *Flashback*

Despite my wife's persistence, she was told again and again that I could not have a transplant due to the high viral load. They could not transplant a patient with this amount of virus in the blood. This reasoning was understandable as there was no need for a new liver in a body plagued with cancer that had spread to the bones, end-stage cirrhosis, and high viral load. The viruses and the cancer would suffocate any new liver I received. I think the delay in having an outright transplant became a disguised blessing. I hoped for a miracle.

Chapter 5

The liver REJUVENATION AND wellness recipes

The philosophy of the liver rejuvenation plan takes into consideration the rhythms of the body. *The 1998 surgeon general's report on nutrition and health concludes that 15 out of every 21 deaths in the United States involve nutrition.* It needs to be reinforced that individuals

"Nutritional deficiency not only is the cause of diseases, but that by correcting the deficiency, disease can not only be prevented but also cured"

Barefoot

with serious health concerns need to work through the rejuvenation plan with a provider that is sympathetic with alternative medicine. Fruits and vegetable juices are part of the rejuvenation program. Diabetics can get the same results if they use vegetable juices instead of fruit juices. The rejuvenation plan is not suitable for pregnant women or those breast-feeding. The aim of the liver rejuvenation plan is to make you have an ageless health, inside out .My opinion about low carbohydrates diets was radically changed after I read the book *Life without Bread*. It describes how low-carbohydrate nutrition can reverse our susceptibility to chronic degenerative diseases.

The Body's Daily Rhythm

From 4 a.m. until 12 noon, the body is in its eliminative phase, having had its last meal the previous evening. This accounts for the "yucky" feeling and the desire to brush your teeth and take a shower in the morning—a desire to eliminate. The body is said to be coming out of a fast, having had its last meal the previous evening. Because the body is eliminating, foods that assist in elimination are encouraged during breakfast. We complete the elimination when we brush our teeth, take a shower, and go to the bathroom. In doing these, we are yielding to a call of nature to finish what it has started. We will introduce you to juices and breakfast recipes that aid elimination. Juices and water are particularly crucial in assisting the elimination process.

From 12 noon until 8 p.m., the body is in a digestion or assimilation phase. Because the body is assimilating nutrients, the first major meals of the day are best taken within this time periods. This is when lunch and dinner are served. The liver rejuvenation plan will introduce you to nutrients that the body will assimilate and use for repair and rejuvenation of the liver.

From 8 p.m. until 4 a.m. the body is in a repair phase. The last meal of the day should be on or before 8 p.m. It is advisable to be in bed by 9 p.m. This is the time when the body utilizes nutrients assimilated for repair and rejuvenation. This is when the hormones are at work building and repairing worn out tissues.

From about 8 p.m., the digestive system begins to shut down and hand over activities to the repair hormones. Any meal taken after this time stays in the stomach for long period of time. Purification, fermentation, indigestion, constipation, and weight gain occur. Eating after 8 p.m. is like throwing a spanner in the wheel of the human body's rhythmic flow. Think what happens to plants that are exposed to sunlight after sunset. In the human body, food will not be digested, and acid reflux will develop.

Alternatives to homemade vegetable juices
We have super foods in the appendix, from powdered ground fruits to vegetables, protein powders, and fibers that will give you the same benefits as juices and salads. Organic aloe vera juices from health food store are also recommended.

Making the transition
- The liver rejuvenation plan will help you lose weight even though it is not the primary rejuvenation plan. Any transition from about 4,000 calories of western diet to about 2,000 calories of whole food will normally cause detoxification, weight loss, and rejuvenation. Please look at the chapter on healing crises to know how to deal with detox reactions.
- Spend about eight weeks with these recipes, and throughout the day drink 6 – 8 eight-ounce glasses of water, spread all through the day.

- Do about 30 – 45 minutes of light aerobic and/or cardiovascular exercise three times a week to help with elimination and circulation. Every action throughout the day should be a form of exercise. Stay active all day.
- Do juice and/or vegetable fasting one day each week during the eight-week period. This can be on an off day. Do not exercise on the fast days, either. Get clarifications from your doctor if you have questions. You can substitute juices with super food formulas mixed with shakes. These can be obtained in a health food store. Looks at the appendix for suggestions.
- We highly recommend you have a liver/gallbladder flush on a fast day, preferably during the third week of the rejuvenation plan. This should coincide with the time you do your first enema or colonic irrigation. Do no physical exercises during a flush. Do another colonic or coffee enema at the eighth week, too.
- We highly recommend small meals during the day instead of the big three. Go slow on the carbohydrates and high on fruits and vegetables and proteins. You can obtain most of your proteins from chicken or eggs, as long as they are free range, sea food, and fish as long as they are not farmed. Other vegetable sources of protein are seeds, legumes, and whole grains.
- We do not recommend pork, red meat, and diary products during the eight-week menu plan.
- If possible have a sauna, foot detox, and lymphatic massage during the third and eighth weeks.
- Cheat occasionally, but do not feel guilty.
- Take your herbs, including milk thistle and any of the bile-moving herbs, daily during the eight-week period and thereafter.
- Look for a health food store in your neighborhood and ask about seminars on healthy living.
- For cooking, use sea salt and rock salt instead of iodized salt, use coconut oil, and olive oil instead of vegetable oils, use filtered water instead of tap water, and use raw honey and unprocessed brown sugar instead of white sugar.

The liver rejuvenation plan aims to shift you from an acidic to an alkaline constitution not by taking you away from what you like to eat but by introducing your favorite dishes in healthy portions. Our diets should be 80 percent alkaline and 20 percent acidic for optimum health. Fruits and vegetable are alkaline, but starches and proteins are acidic. We also recommend at least 40 percent of the food you eat while on this program be raw and from fruits and vegetables to supply the needed pro-biotics, fibers, enzymes, antioxidants, and chelating agents the liver needs to eliminate toxins, heal, and regenerate. We emphasize poultry and sea foods over red meat in this plan, too.

The liver regeneration food plan encourages small meals spread over the day because large meals put undue strain on the liver and the digestive system. Also, the energy reserves of the body are directed to the digestive system, which creates imbalances and deficiencies in the energy demand of other organ systems.

We aim to introduce you to varieties of food, because eating one particular food in excess creates deficiencies in other food groups, which defeat the purpose of the liver rejuvenation health plan. In preparing for the food plan, I advice that you work to end your addictions to caffeine, sweeteners, tobacco, and alcohol. Be aware of the withdrawal reactions, too.

For individuals with weak constitutions, end-stages liver disease, acid reflux, and digestion problems, it is advisable to combine foods wisely in a manner that prevents additional strain on the digestive system. Since fruits, vegetables, and melons digest faster with less effort from the digestive system, it is advisable to wait before eating them with carbohydrates and proteins that put more demands on the digestive system. We aim to introduce you to menu plans that will not hold foods up in the stomach any longer than necessary. This prevents putrefaction and makes it possible to eliminate within 12 – 18 hours of eating, as nature intended. We want to be sure that the foods we eat at dinner are out of our body by the time we are having lunch the next day. Eating nutritious foods in the best possible combination is crucial to the rejuvenation of the liver and to re-establishing our energy level and to ensuring that there are two bowel movements daily. We present this program as a guide and not a rule. We want you to be flexible with yourself in choosing the best combinations you desire.

We recommend eating melons alone because they are digested very quickly. Eating melons with other foods can hold up its digestion. Since it digests easily, it can ferment and cause gaseous putrefaction and decomposition if left to hang around for too long in the stomach. Also, the fermentation leads to the production of alcohol in the digestive tract.

Starches do not combine well with meats, so meats should be eaten with rice, potatoes, or bread. This is because the stomach produces hydrochloric acid to digest the meat, which is neutralized by the alkaline juices the stomach produces to digest starches. Consequently, both the carbohydrates and the meats are undigested and they stay in the stomach for a longer period of time, causing purification, gas, and auto-intoxification.

We recommend eating the salads before the regular meals because fruits and vegetables are digested before starches and proteins. Eating salads with starches and proteins can hold them longer than necessary in the stomach. Like the other scenarios, these can lead to decomposition and fermentation.

The fermentation, putrefaction, gas, bad breath, indigestion, and acid reflux are conventionally managed with antacids. What antacids do is to antagonize the acid gas generated from improper food combinations and indigestion in the stomach that contribute to the discomfort felt by most people. Through biofeedback mechanisms, the brain notices the absence of acid in the stomach and stimulates the productions of copious amounts of hydrochloric acid that was neutralized by the presence of starches in a portentous diet. To alleviate this problem, we recommend separating high proteins from starches and/or addition of lemon or lime juice to our water to supply the needed acid the digestive system needs.

We will introduce you to lifestyles, foods, and remedies that will aid detoxification, re-mineralization, and regeneration. As Dr Henry Lindlahr puts it, *'To seek to kill germs without purifying and invigorating the organism would be like trying to keep a house free from fungi and vermin by sprinkling it daily with carbonic acid and other germ killers instead of flooding it with fresh air and sunshine and washing it out thoroughly. The antiseptic would only add to the filth.'* Most likely, those just starting the plan will have a need to detoxify themselves of accumulated wastes in their blood and organs. We will introduce nutrients and herbs that will facilitate the process. We want you to be aware of some of the forms of detox reactions, too. If these occur, please refer to the chapter on healing reactions to learn how to deal with them.

Be kind to yourself. You can take a day off now and then and be your usual self. If you miss a particular section, just skip it and keep going. It is a lifestyle you are acquiring and not just an eight-week program. Your metabolism should be firing up, and you will probably be eliminating more toxins.

Breakfast
- Upon rising, we highly recommend about 10 minutes of meditation and reflection.
- If you prefer doing your exercises instead, exercise for about 25 minutes.
- Take a glass of water followed by fresh fruit or vegetable juice to aid the eliminative phase of your body rhythm. You can use the super food formulas as smoothies or protein drinks in place of juicing. You can also take an herbal tea of your choice, preferably green tea, lemon tea, black tea, or ginger tea.
- Takes your break fast from the breakfast recipe along with your vitamins, herb and medicines

Lunch
- Take you lunch from the chosen recipes.
- Please pray before having your lunch.
- Take your medicines, vitamins, and/or herbs before or after lunch, as prescribed.

Dinner
- Pray.
- Take your dinner from the recipes.
- Take your medicines and supplements before or after dinner as prescribed. Take your vegetable juices or super food formula.
- Don't be a couch potato after dinner. Exercise if you did not exercise in the morning, or engage in some form of light physical activity to help digestion for about 15 minutes.

- You may take valerian or chamomile tea to relax your muscles and to aid sleep.
- Go to bed by 9 p.m.

The Recipes

We do not want to be your food police but to present you with the recipes and let you make your selection because we respect choices. As the legendry musician James Brown put it 'open the door for me and I will go and get what I want myself'

Our chef has meticulously prepared the menus included in the liver regeneration food plans. As a culinary consultant, she has helped thousands of people make food choices that fit their lifestyles, while maximizing the health benefits of foods. She helps individuals in supporting healthy dietary habits and making the transition from the standard American diet to healthier dietary lifestyles, while breaking out from the "food rut." She says, just like a car, the body needs top quality fuels to operate at peak levels. Here is how she puts it: "Food is fuel for the body and your life. Regular assessment of that fuel is necessary to see if the food you are eating is actually working for or against you. What do you eat? When do you eat? How much of it do you eat it? And how do all of these factors improve your health, vitality, and your overall performance. Food isn't just what you eat. It affects how you feel. As a chef, I can optimize your diet so that you get the best fuel for your life."

Food is fun, and changing your relationship with food can literally save your life. Fad diets are unhealthy, but in order to make permanent health changes to your diet, you may need all the support you need. Quick fixes and sudden rapid changes can be detrimental to your body, and actually reverse the benefits of dietary changes. The recipes in the liver rejuvenation food plans will help you make a dietary shift by supplying you with healthier portions of your food choices while supplying you with appropriate recipes,.

The Environmental Working Group publishes a list of the 12 fruits and vegetables with the most and least pesticide residues. Their 2003 survey found that nectarines, pears, and peaches had the most pesticides, while broccoli and peas had low amounts of such toxins.

Twelve Fruits and Vegetables with The Most Pesticide Residues

Apples	Bell Peppers
Celery	Cherries
Imported Grapes	Nectarines
Peaches	Pears
Potatoes	Red Raspberries
Spinach	Strawberries

Twelve Fruits and Vegetables with the least pesticide residues

Asparagus	Avocados
Bananas	Broccoli
Cauliflowers	Corn (Sweet)
Kiwi	Mangos
Onions	Papaya
Pineapples	Peas (Sweet)

Breakfast
Apple Oatmeal Pancakes
Makes 8 pancakes.
- 2 tablespoons oats
- 2 teaspoons oat bran
- 3/4 cup whole wheat flour
- 1/2 teaspoon cinnamon
- 2 teaspoons baking powder
- 1/4 teaspoon salt
- 1/2 cup unsweetened apple sauce

Combine the oats, oat bran, wheat flour, cinnamon, baking powder, and salt. Stir in the apple sauce until dry ingredients are completely moistened. If the mixture seems stiff, add unsweetened apple juice or water until the consistency is smooth. To cook, pour ¼ cup of onto a lightly oiled skillet or griddle over medium-high heat. Cook until bottom is brown and spatula slips easily underneath. Turn and brown other side.

Cranberry Peach Compote
- 1 1/4 ounce bag of frozen peaches
- ½ cup dried cranberries
- 2 tablespoons of honey or unrefined sugar
- 2 tablespoons of water

Combine ingredients in a medium size saucepan. Simmer gently over medium-low heat, stirring occasionally until the mixture is bubbly and begins to thicken, about 15 minutes. Serve over pancakes.

Scrambled Eggs with Smoked Salmon and Dill
Serves 3.
- 6 large eggs
- 1/2 tablespoon fresh dill, minced
- 4 ounces smoked salmon
- 2 tablespoons oil
- sea or rock salt and pepper to taste

Crack eggs into a large bowl and beat with a fork or whisk until fluffy. Add dill, and season with salt and pepper. Heat 2 teaspoons of oil in a large skillet over medium-high heat. Pour in the egg mixture and cook for about 4 minutes or until the mixture starts to set. Stir in pieces of smoked salmon, and continue cooking for another 1 – 3 minutes until eggs reach desired firmness.

Breakfast Burrito with Turkey Sausage and Salsa
Makes 4 burritos.
- 1/4 pound turkey sausage, cubed
- ½ medium onion, diced
- ½ medium tomato, diced
- 1 garlic clove, minced
- 2 eggs, beaten lightly
- 4 10-inch multi-grain tortillas

Heat 2 teaspoons of oil in a pan over medium high heat. Add onion and cook until onions begin to turn translucent. Add garlic, tomato, and sausage. Cook for 5 – 10 minutes. Add eggs, stirring occasionally until the eggs are set. Spoon mixture down the center of warm tortillas and roll to form burritos. Top with salsa if desired.

Mushroom and Vegetable Frittata
Serves 4.

- 6 eggs
- 1/2 medium onion, diced
- ½ medium bell pepper, diced
- ½ large zucchini, diced
- ½ cup broccoli, chopped
- ½ cup mushrooms, cut into bite sized pieces
- salt and pepper to taste

Preheat the oven to 350°F. Heat 2 teaspoons of oil in an oven-proof pan over medium-high heat. Add the vegetables until they are tender, about 6 – 10 minutes. Meanwhile, crack the eggs into a large bowl and beat with a whisk or fork. Season with salt and pepper. When vegetables are tender, pour in the egg mixture tilting the pan to distribute eggs evenly throughout. Reduce the heat to medium and cook on the stove top for 5 more minutes or until eggs begin to set. Transfer the pan to the oven. Bake in the oven until the top of the frittata is set, about 10 – 15 minutes. Slice the frittata into wedges and serve.

Cinnamon Oatmeal with Apricots and Almonds
Serves 4.
- 3 cups water
- 2 cups old-fashioned oats
- 1 teaspoon salt
- 1 cup unsweetened apple juice
- 1 cup apricots, sliced
- 1/4 cup golden brown sugar, packed
- 1/4 cup toasted almonds
- 1/2 teaspoon powdered cinnamon

Bring 3 cups of water to a boil in a medium saucepan. Add oats and salt and stir over medium heat until oats are softened, about 5 minutes. As the oatmeal thickens, add the apple juice, chopped apricots, brown sugar, almonds, and cinnamon. Reduce heat to low, cover and continue cooking about 5 minutes.

Spiced Sweet Potato Hash
Serves 2.
- 1/4 pound turkey sausage, cubed
- 1 medium sweet potato, dice one large red onion, thinly sliced, divided
- ½ medium onion, diced
- ½ medium bell pepper, diced

- 2 teaspoons chili powder
- 1 teaspoon ground cumin
- 1/2 teaspoon of turmeric
- 1 teaspoons ground cinnamon
- sea or rock salt and pepper to taste

Heat 2 teaspoons of oil in a pan over medium heat. Add the sausage and cook until mostly done, about 5 minutes. Add the sweet potato, onion, and bell pepper. Season with chili powder, cumin, turmeric, and cinnamon. Stir frequently and continue cooking until the potatoes are tender, about 10 minutes. Add fresh parsley or cilantro if desired.

The Soups
Hearty Mushroom Barley Soup
Serves 4.

- 1/4 cup barley
- 1 large onion, diced
- 2 ribs of celery, diced
- 1 pound mixed mushroom, thickly chopped
- ½ cup tomato sauce
- 16 ounces vegetable, chicken, or beef broth or water.
- 2 medium carrots, diced
- ½ cup fresh parsley leaves, roughly chopped
- sea or rock salt and pepper to taste

In a medium saucepan, bring 2 cups of water to a boil and add barley. Cover and reduce heat to medium, simmering until the barely is tender, about 20 minutes. Drain the barely and set it aside. Meanwhile, in a large pot, heat 2 teaspoons of oil over medium-high heat. Add onions, celery and carrots, stirring occasionally until onions are tender, about 5 – 7 minutes. Add mushrooms, carrots, and celery, and cook for another five minutes or until the mushrooms begin to brown. Add tomato sauce, 3 cups of water, and barley. Season with salt and pepper. Simmer 15 minutes, stir in fresh parsley, cook for 5 more minutes, and serve.

Sweet Corn, Spinach and Crab Soup
Serves 4.

- 1 cup sweet corn kernels
- ½ medium onion, diced
- 1 garlic clove, minced
- 1 cup spinach leaves

- 3 cups fish or water stock
- 1 6-ounce can of crabmeat, drained and flaked
- sea or rock salt and pepper to taste

Heat 2 teaspoons of oil in a saucepan over medium-high heat. Add onions and cook until they turn translucent, about 5 minutes. Add the corn and garlic and cook for about 2 minutes. Add in the fish stock or water, and season with salt and pepper. Simmer over medium-low heat for 5 minutes. Add crabmeat and spinach simmer for 2-5 minutes and serve.

Spanish Fish and Shrimp Stew
Serves: 4.
- 1 pound each of wild-raised cod and snapper fillet, cut into chunks
- 12 medium wild-raised shrimp
- 1/4 cup olive oil
- 1 large onion, diced
- 1 15-ounce can diced stewed tomatoes
- 3 cloves garlic, minced
- 1/2 teaspoon saffron or paprika
- ½ cup fresh parsley leaves
- 3 cups fish stock or water
- sea or rock salt and pepper to taste

In a heavy large pot, heat 2 teaspoons of oil over medium high heat. Add onion and cook until it becomes translucent. Add the tomatoes, garlic, saffron, or paprika and fish stock or water and bring up to a boil. Reduce heat to medium, season with salt and pepper, add fish and simmer for15 minutes. Add parsley just before serving.

Coconut Chicken and Mushroom Soup
Serves 4.
- 1 pound free-range chicken, cut into chunks or thinly sliced
- 2 14 oz. cans coconut milk
- 2 cups water
- 1 inch of ginger root, peeled and grated
- 1/4 cup lime juice
- 1 teaspoon cayenne pepper
- 1/2 teaspoon ground turmeric
- 2 green onions (scallions), sliced thinly
- ¼ cup fresh cilantro leaves

- sea or rock salt and pepper to taste

In a large pot, heat 2 teaspoons of oil over medium-high heat. Add chicken and cook until the chicken turns white, about 5 minutes. Add coconut milk and water and bring up to a bottle. Reduce to medium heat, season with salt, cayenne, and turmeric. Simmer for another 10 – 15 minutes or until the chicken is done. Add green onions and cilantro just before serving.

Indian Split Peas and Spinach Soup
Serves 4.
- 1 medium onion, diced
- 3 garlic cloves, minced
- 3 large tomatoes, chopped
- 2 cups fresh spinach leaves
- 1 cup green slit peas
- 1 inch of ginger, peeled and grated
- 1 teaspoon chili powder
- 1 teaspoon ground turmeric
- 1 teaspoon ground cumin
- 1 tablespoon lemon juice
- sea or rock salt and pepper to taste

Add split peas to a small saucepan and cover with one inch of water. Bring to a boil, remove from heat, and let soak for 15 minutes. Drain the water and reserve. Meanwhile, in a large pot, heat 2 teaspoons of oil over medium-high heat. Add onions and garlic and cook until tender. Add tomatoes, cover the pot and let simmer until the tomatoes are soft, about 5 – 7 minutes, then mash the tomatoes in the pan with a spatula. Add split peas and season with chili, turmeric, cumin, and salt. Add 4 cups of water, then stir and simmer over medium heat for about 15 minutes. Add the spinach and lemon juice and simmer for 10 more minutes or until the split peas are done and have begun to disintegrate.

Sausage, Kale and White Bean Soup
Serves 4.
- 1 cans white beans (Great Northern, cannellini, or navy beans)
- 1 medium onions, diced
- 2 garlic cloves, minced
- 2 1/2 cups chicken broth

- 1 bay leaf
- 1/2 pound turkey sausage, diced
- 3 carrots, diced
- ½ pound kale, coarsely chopped
- 2 tablespoons parsley, coarsely chopped
- sea or rock salt and pepper to taste

Drain beans into a colander and rinse. In a large pot cook onions and sausage in 2 teaspoons of oil over medium high heat for about 5 minutes. Add garlic and cook for a minute longer, while stirring. Add beans, broth, 2 cups of water, salt, pepper, carrots and bay leaf, and simmer, uncovered for about 20 minutes. Add kale, 2 cups of water and simmer until the kale is tender, about 10 to 15 minutes, stirring occasionally. Remove and discard bay leaf before serving. Garnish with fresh chopped parsley.

The Snacks
Pizza Bread
Serves 3.
- 1/2 whole wheat baguette (sliced) or 6 slices of whole wheat bread
- 6 ounces of low fat mozzarella, shredded
- 1 16-ounce jar pasta sauce
- 1 1/2 tablespoon. dried Italian herb blend

Toast bread under broiler until lightly browned, about 5 minutes. Top with 2 tablespoons of pasta sauce, and sprinkle on herbs and cheese on each half. Broil again about 1 to 2 minutes or until cheese is melted.

Fruit Kabobs with Yogurt Dip
- ½ cup cantaloupe melon, peeled and chunked
- 1/2 cup honeydew melon, peeled and chunked
- 1/2 cup small strawberries, whole
- ½ cup pineapple chunks
- 2 small bananas, peeled and cut into 1 inch chunks
- 1 – 2 tablespoons cup orange juice
- juice from 1 lime
- 1 8-ounce container of vanilla low-fat yogurt
- 2 tablespoons ground cinnamon

Alternately skewer cantaloupe, honeydew, strawberries, pineapple, and bananas onto kabobs. Place into a shallow pan. Combine orange and lime juice and pour over kabobs. Chill 30 – 60 minutes. In a bowl, combine yogurt and 2 tablespoons of orange juice. Cover and chill. To serve, place kabobs onto a platter, discarding juice mixture. Sprinkle with cinnamon and serve with yogurt dip.

Hummus

- 2 cloves garlic, minced
- ¼ cup lemon juice
- ¼ cup water
- 14-ounce can chickpeas (garbanzo beans), rinsed and drained
- ½ cup tahini paste
- 1 teaspoon sea salt

Place all ingredients in a food processor or blender and process until smooth, scraping the sides occasionally, and adding olive oil if more liquid is needed.

Spinach Dip

8 servings.

- ¼ cup non-fat plain yogurt
- 1 tablespoon lemon juice
- 1 tablespoon water
- 1 clove of garlic, minced
- ½ teaspoon dried Italian herb blend
- 1 cup of chopped fresh spinach leaves

Combine ingredients, except spinach, in a food processor or blender and process until smooth. Pour into a bowl, stir in spinach and chill for from one hour up to overnight. Stir and serve with fresh vegetables for dipping.

Strawberry Banana Smoothie

Serves 3.

- 1 ½ cups vanilla yogurt
- 10 ounces frozen strawberries
- 1 medium banana sliced
- ¼ cup unsweetened apple juice

Combine all ingredients in a blender, processing until smooth, and scraping down the sides as necessary. Serve immediately.

Baked Sweet Potato Chips

- 1 medium sweet potato, peeled and sliced into thin rounds

- 2 tablespoons olive oil
- ½ teaspoon cinnamon
- ½ teaspoon cayenne pepper
- sea or rock salt to taste

Heat oven to 350°F. Peel sweet potato and slice thin, as if for a thick potato chip. Place potato slices into a bowl, toss with oil and spices. Spread evenly on a non-stick baking sheet, bake for 20 minutes, turn and bake for another 10 minutes.

The Salads
Turkey Strawberry and Walnut Spinach Salad
Serves 4.
- 1 pound fresh spinach
- 1 pint strawberries, halved
- 1/2 cup walnuts, toasted
- 6 slices of deli turkey, cut into 2 inch wide strips

Place clean spinach in a large bowl. Wrap strawberries in the turkey strips and add to the spinach. Top with toasted walnuts. Toss with poppy seed vinaigrette.

Poppy Seed Vinaigrette
- 1/3 cup raspberry vinegar
- 1 teaspoon Dijon mustard
- 1/2 cup of honey
- 1 cup olive oil
- 1 1/2 tablespoons poppy seeds
- ½ teaspoon of sea salt

Except for the olive oil, place all of the ingredients in a bowl. Mix together with a whisk, then, while whisking, drizzle in the olive oil.

Three Melon and Mint Salad
Serves 4.
- 3 cups thinly sliced melon (honeydew, cantaloupe, watermelon, etc.)
- 2 tablespoons lime juice
- 1 tablespoon chopped fresh mint leaves
- 2 tablespoons honey

Combine melons, lime juice, mint, and honey in a glass or plastic bowl. Refrigerate and allow marinating for two hours before serving. Serve at room temperature.

Mediterranean Albacore Tuna Salad
Serves 4.
- 2 cans tuna, marinated and packed in olive oil
- 1 green onion (scallion), thinly sliced
- 4 large black olives, chopped
- 2 teaspoons red wine vinegar
- 2 tablespoons capers, drained and rinsed
- 1 clove garlic, minced
- 2 teaspoons lemon juice of one lemon
- 2 tablespoons pine nuts
- ½ lb. spinach
- ½ lb. mixed salad greens
- 1/8 cup fresh parsley leaves
- 1 cup of mixed sprouts (alfalfa, radish, broccoli, mung bean)

Drain and combine the tuna with green onion, olives, vinegar, capers, garlic, and lemon juice. Refrigerate and let marinate for at least 2 hours. Toss together spinach, mixed salad greens, parsley, and sprouts in a bowl. Top with tuna mixture. Sprinkle with pine nuts.

Hummus Salad Wrap
Makes 2 wraps.
- 2 10-inch multi-grain tortillas
- ¼ cup hummus
- 1 cup lettuce, chopped
- ½ cup cucumbers, sliced
- ½ tomato, chopped
- 8 large pitted olives, halved
- 2 tablespoons light Italian dressing
- ¼ cup alfalfa sprouts

Spread hummus down the center of the tortillas. Top with lettuce, and then top the lettuce with all remaining ingredients. Drizzle dressing over the salad, and then roll up the wrap.

Curried Chicken Salad

Serves 4.

- 2 cups cooked free-range chicken, cubed, sliced, or shredded
- 8 ounces mandarin oranges, drained
- 1 cup seedless grapes, halved
- 8 ounces pineapple chunks, drained
- ½ cup celery, diced
- ½ cup plain non-fat yogurt
- 1 teaspoon curry powder
- 1/2 teaspoon turmeric
- 1 teaspoon lemon juice
- ¼ teaspoon ground ginger
- 1 pound mixed salad greens
- sea or rock salt and pepper to taste

Mix chicken, celery, oranges, grapes, and pineapple. Mix mayonnaise, curry powder, salt, pepper, turmeric, and ginger. Gently stir into chicken mixture. Refrigerate at least 2 hours. Spoon onto mixed salad greens salad greens.

The Desserts
Raspberry Apple Crisp
Serves 4.

- ¼ pound Granny Smith apples
- 1 1/4 cups fresh raspberries
- 2 tablespoons brown sugar
- 1 – 2 teaspoon ground cinnamon
- 2 tablespoons lemon juice
- 2 tablespoons whole-wheat flour
- 2/3 cups rolled oats
- 1/8 cup olive oil

Preheat oven to 350°F. Peel, core, and slice the apples. In a bowl, combine apple slices, raspberries, brown sugar, cinnamon, and lemon juice. Pour into a baking dish. In another bowl, combine flour, oats and oil, mixing well. Top the fruit mixture with the oat topping. Bake for 40 minutes or until the top is golden brown and bubbling.

Tangerines with Pistachios
Serves 4.

- 5 tangerines, peeled and segmented
- 1 tablespoon brown sugar
- ¼ cup of orange juice

- 1 tablespoon chopped pistachios

Place tangerine segments in a wide shallow dish. In a bowl, combine sugar, and orange juice. Pour the juice mixture over the fruit and let chill in the refrigerator for at least an hour. Mix the dish prior to serving and top with pistachios.

Peach and Yogurt Parfait

Serves 2.
- 1 peach, diced
- 1 cup of granola with nuts
- 2/3 cup low fat plain yogurt
- 1 tablespoon of fruit juice
- 1 tablespoon all natural preserved fruit

In two parfait or tall glasses, evenly distribute the fruit. Top each layer with granola, and top granola with yogurt. Combine the juice and jam in a small bowl. Drizzle over the yogurt.

Oat Crisps

Makes one dozen or more.
- 1 3/4 cups of rolled oats
- ½ cup brown sugar
- 1 egg
- 4 tablespoons oil
- 2 tablespoons maple or vanilla extract

Preheat oven to 375°F.

Mix oats and sugar in a bowl with egg, oil, and maple or vanilla extract. Let sit for 15 minutes.

Place 1 teaspoon of the mixture at a time onto a lightly oiled baking sheet about 2 inches apart. With the back of a fork, press each mound into a round 3-inch disc. Bake 10 – 15 minutes, let cool and remove from baking sheet.

Brownies

- 10 ounces applesauce
- 8 ounces cocoa powder or melted dark chocolate
- 1/4 teaspoon sea salt
- 2 cups sugar brown or unrefined sugar
- 1 banana, mashed with a fork
- 1 1/3 cups finely ground whole wheat flour

- 2 cups vegan chocolate chips or dark chocolate chips

Combine all ingredients until smooth. Transfer into a square 8-inch by 8-inch or similar baking pan. Bake at 350°F for 35 minutes. Allow to cool for 10 minutes before removing from the pan.

Banana Cake

Serves 8.

- 2 cups unbleached all-purpose or whole wheat pastry flour
- 1 1/2 teaspoons baking soda
- 1/2 teaspoon sea or rock salt
- 1 cup raw sugar, brown sugar, or other natural sweetener
- 1/3 cup oil
- 4 ripe bananas
- 1/4 cup water
- 1 teaspoon vanilla extract
- 1 cup chopped walnuts

Preheat oven to 350°F. Mix flour, baking soda, and salt in a bowl. In a large bowl, beat sugar and oil together, then add the bananas and mash them. Stir in the water and vanilla, and mix thoroughly. Add the flour mixture along with the chopped walnuts, and stir thoroughly. Spread in a non-stick or lightly oil-sprayed 9-inch square baking pan. Bake for 45 – 50 minutes, or until a toothpick inserted into the center comes out clean.

The Poultry Dishes Herb-roasted Cornish hens

Serves 3.

- 2 free-range Cornish hens
- 2 tablespoons poultry seasoning
- 2 tablespoons dried thyme
- 2 tablespoons dried marjoram leaves
- 2 tablespoons dried oregano
- 2 tablespoons garlic powder
- 2 tablespoons onion powder
- 2 tablespoons sea or rock salt

Combine all ingredients except the Cornish hens, adding just enough olive oil to make 2 – 4 tablespoons of paste. Rub the spice blend all over each hen, including inside the body cavity. Tuck the wings under the shoulders and place each hen on its back on a drip pan in a shallow roasting pan. Bake at 350°F for 1 hour 15 minutes or until the juices run clear when you pierce the joint between the thigh and the drumstick.

Spinach and Pine nut Stuffed Chicken Breast
Serves 3.
- 3 free-range chicken breast halves, skinned, boned
- 1/4 cup toasted pine nuts (pignoli)
- 3 cups spinach leaves
- ½ cup cooked brown rice
- 1/2 medium onion, diced
- 1 garlic clove, minced
- sea or rock salt and black pepper to taste

Preheat oven to 350 degrees F. Place one chicken breast half, boned side up, between 2 pieces of plastic wrap or waxed paper. Working from center, gently pound chicken with rolling pin or flat side of meat mallet until about 1/4-inch thick. Repeat with remaining chicken breast halves.

Heat 1 – 2 tablespoons of olive oil medium high heat in a skillet. Add onions and cook until translucent, about 5 minutes. Add garlic, cook for 3 minutes, and then add rice and spinach. Season with salt and pepper and cook until spinach is wilted. Remove from heat and stir in the pine nuts. Place 1/3 cup of spinach mixture down the center third of each chicken breast. Bring the ends of the breasts over stuffing. Fold in the sides. Secure with wooden tooth picks. Place stuffed chicken breasts, seam side down, in an ungreased baking dish. Bake at 350°F for 35 – 40 minutes or until chicken is fork tender and juices run clear.

Turkey Burgers
Serves 4-6.
- 1 pound ground turkey
- ¼ cup Worcestershire sauce
- 1 1/2 teaspoons Dijon-style mustard
- 1 cup quick or old-fashioned oats, uncooked
- ½ medium onion, finely diced
- sea or rock salt and black pepper to taste
- 4 multi-grain or whole wheat burger buns, toasted

Combine all ingredients, except the buns, mixing well. Shape the burgers into patties about the size of your palm and about ½ inch thick. Place on a broil pan and broil 7 – 9 minutes on each side. Serve with desired garnish on toasted buns.

Island Curry Chicken

Serves 4.
- 1 free-range chicken, quartered and skinned
- 1/4 cup fresh thyme
- 1 medium onion, diced
- 5 tablespoons yellow Jamaican curry powder
- 2 cloves garlic, minced
- 3 tablespoons black pepper
- 1 tablespoons chicken seasoning
- Juice from 1 lemon
- 1/2 Scotch Bonnet or Habanero pepper
- 2 medium sweet potatoes, peeled and cubes

Season chicken with all of the herbs and spices and let marinate in the refrigerator for 30 minutes to 24 hours. Season with sea or rock salt and place chicken in a pot with 2 cups of water, bring to a boil, stir, and simmer over medium heat for 20 minutes. Add sweet potatoes and cook until sweet potatoes are tender, about 15 minutes.

Tropical Fruit Chicken Wings
Serves 4.
- 1 dozen chicken wings
- 1 teaspoon each of cumin and turmeric
- 1 teaspoon ground ginger
- 1 8-ounce can pineapple, drained
- 1 firm mango, peeled and sliced
- 1 8-ounce can mandarin orange, drained
- 1 cup seedless grapes, halved

Preheat oven to 350°F. In a bowl, mix together cumin, turmeric, ginger, and sea or rock salt. Add wings, and toss until coated. Transfer wings to a baking dish. In another bowl combine pineapple, mango, oranges and grapes. Pour over chicken, and bake wings for approximately 15 – 20 minutes, turning wings half-way through.

Baked Italian Chicken Breast
Serves 4.
- 4 boneless skinless free-range chicken breasts, halved
- ¼ cup Italian dressing
- 1/4 olive oil
- 1 cup marinara sauce

Preheat oven to 350°F. Place chicken in a large bowl and drizzle with enough olive oil to just coat it. Season with sea or rock salt and black pepper. Coat thoroughly with bread crumbs. Place chicken on a non-stick baking sheet and drizzle with Italian dressing. Bake for 20 minutes, then turn each breast over, add marinara sauce, and continue baking for another 25 minutes or until chicken is cooked through.

Seafood
Spicy Peppered Shrimp
Serves 4.

"Health begins on the farm and not in the pharmacy."
Uncle of Dr Alan Gaby

- 1 1/2 pounds shrimp
- 2 tablespoons olive oil
- 2 cloves garlic, garlic
- 2 tablespoons black pepper
- 2 tablespoons crushed red pepper flake
- ½ teaspoon paprika
- ½ teaspoon turmeric
- sea or rock salt

Preheat oven to 425°F. Heat the oil in a saucepan over medium heat, add the garlic, and cook 3 –4 minutes. Remove from heat; add salt, pepper, red pepper flake, paprika, and turmeric, stirring to mix. Toss shrimp in spice mixture and pour into a shallow baking dish. Bake until the shrimp turn pink and opaque, about 10 minutes, stirring once to turn the shrimp over.

Moroccan Salmon

2 servings.

- 2 tablespoons cilantro leaves, chopped
- 2 tablespoons parsley, chopped
- 2 teaspoons fresh lime juice
- ½ teaspoon garlic, minced
- ½ teaspoon extra virgin olive oil
- ¼ teaspoon cumin
- ¼ teaspoon turmeric
- 1/4 teaspoon paprika
- ¼ teaspoon chili powder
- 2 6-ounce salmon fillets
- sea or rock salt and pepper to taste

Place salmon fillets in a shallow glass baking dish or plate. In a medium bowl, combine all ingredients, except the salmon, stirring to make a paste. Rub the paste evenly over the salmon. Refrigerate 15 minutes to 2 hours. Heat 2 teaspoons of oil in a pan over medium high heat. Carefully add salmon, cooking 2 minutes on each side. Continue cooking 6 – 9 minutes or until fish flakes easily with a fork or reaches desired doneness.

Red Snapper Escovitch

2 servings.

- 6oz. red snapper fillets
- 1 red bell pepper, sliced into strips
- 1 medium onion, sliced into strips
- 1 medium carrot, sliced into strips
- 1 inch peeled ginger, grated
- 2 cloves garlic, minced
- 1 tablespoon fresh cilantro, chopped
- 2 tablespoons fresh lime juice
- sea or rock salt and pepper to taste

Season the fish with salt and pepper. Heat oil in a pan over medium high heat. Carefully add the fish and cook for 4 minutes before turning over. Add lime juice, garlic, ginger, carrots, onions, and bell pepper around the fish. Top with cilantro, cover, and cook over medium-low heat for 6 –10 minutes or until fish is flaky and white.

Crispy Baked Tilapia Tacos

Makes 4 tacos.

- 4 3-ounce tilapia fillets
- 1 egg, beaten
- 1/2 cup seasoned Panko breadcrumbs
- 4 six-inch multi grain tortillas
- 1 cup cabbage, thinly sliced
- ½ cup fresh cilantro

Preheat oven to 450°F. Pat fish dry, season with salt, pepper and cumin. Submerge fillets in beaten egg and dredge through the bread crumbs. Dip the fillets back into the egg, and dredge through the breadcrumbs again. Bake in a 450°F oven for 5 minutes, turn over and cook for 5 more minutes. Place each fillet on a tortilla, top with cabbage, cilantro leaves, and white sauce (below).

White Sauce

- 1/2 cup plain non-fat yogurt
- 2 tablespoons lime juice
- 1 tablespoon jalapeno pepper, minced
- 1 teaspoon capers
- 1/2 teaspoon dried oregano
- 1/2 teaspoon ground cumin
- 1 teaspoon cayenne pepper

Combine all the ingredients gradually, adding lime juice so as not to make it too thin.

Baked Fish with Lemon and Thyme

Serves 4.

- 1 ½ lbs fish fillets
- ½ cup lemon juice
- ½ teaspoon dried thyme
- 2 tablespoon olive oil

Combine lemon juice, salt, pepper, and thyme in a shallow dish. Add fish and turn to coat. Cover and refrigerate for at least 30 minutes, turning occasionally. Drain fish, brush with olive oil, and place on a shallow pan and bake until the fish is opaque throughout and flakes with a fork.

Understanding food labels

Since 2002, organic produce in the United States has been specially labeled. Organic-certified production forbids genetically modified organisms and irradiation as well as the use of sewage sludge, herbicides, insecticides, and pesticides. To qualify as a certified organic farmer, a farmer must certify that they have forgone soil-rescue chemicals for at least three years, promoted soil health by employing soil building, and have used conservation practices, manure management, and crop rotation. Organic livestock must eats only organic feeds, and have outdoor access to pasture land.

- A "100-percent" organic label means that the product has 100 percent organic ingredients.
- A "simply-organic" label means between 95 – 100 percent of the ingredients are organic.
- A "made with organic ingredients" label means at least 70 percent of the ingredients are organic.
- "Natural" means less than 70 percent of the ingredients are organic.
- "Not from concentrate" means no additives or filler are added.
- For information on non-profit organic volunteers, ages 16 – 65, with organic farm experience who have worked on about 1,100 farms in America and Lain American countries, visit www. GrowFood.org, or the worldwide opportunities for organic farming at www.wwoof.com.
- For a wallet-sized guide about pesticides in your produce, visit www.foodnews.org.
- To find a farm or farmer with fresh produce in your community visit www.CSA-center.org.
- To learn more about the impact of industrial farming on the environment, visit www.sustainabletable.org.
- To get involved in an organic consumers association to maintain the standards of organics in the face of attempts to dilute those standards, visit www.organicconsumer.org or www.cornucopia.org.
- Typical produce is often jet-lagged and weary after traveling hundreds or thousands of miles to your grocery stores. To find

the country of origin or region of the country of your produce, visit www.foodroutes.org.

Dietary Modifications for the Ailing Liver

Modern life has progressed to the point where foods are chemically fertilized, sprayed for bugs, preserved for shelf life and enhanced for flavor. The lifeless end-product is re-enriched with artificial vitamins and synthetic minerals. After years of consuming such foods, our bodies become artificial and react to those chemicals by manifesting them as disease. Conventional medicine responds with more synthetic drugs to sustain our lives.

Because humans were biologically predisposed to feed directly from the soil, there is interdependence between the human and soil ecosystems. Disruptions in either one adversely affects human or plant life. In the early 1930s, Harvard-trained dentist Dr. Weston Price, traveled the world and extensively researched the role of nutrition in physical degeneration and the causes and consequences of food adulteration. He found that in primitive cultures where people lived close to the soil, physical and organ degeneration were minimal when compared to Western cultures where the consumption of foods correlates to degenerative diseases and predispositions to infections.

Two-times Nobel Laureate Dr. Linus Pauling corroborated this view when he indicated that our ability to manufacture vitamins was discarded at a time when our ancestors lived in close proximity to fruits and vegetables and did not need to produce them within themselves. With evolution, industrialization, and modernization, they moved from fruit and vegetables habitats to more organized settlements and suffered great vitamin deficiencies. He believed these nutritional deficiencies, coupled with modernized farming, inadequate supplementation, and aquaculture have led to the proliferation of deficiency and many of the diseases in modern man.

In addition to antioxidants and vitamins, sterols and sterolins were processed out of foods as the evolutionary trends continued. These substances are nature's armor and breast plate against organ degeneration and infections. They are phytonutrients (secondary compounds) referred to as "plant fat", or phytosterols, and were discovered in 1922. They are vital components of plants are found in whole, raw, and unprocessed fruits, vegetables, seed, nuts, cereals, legumes, and soy products. While humans use and make the good cholesterols, plants use the phytosterols. They have anti-inflammatory and immuno-modulatory functions. In chronic inflammatory liver diseases, sterols and sterolins were found to arrest the destruction of liver cells and stop progression to cancer by normalizing the level of inflammatory messengers like interleukin-6, the major player in chronic inflammatory diseases, controlling liver inflammations, and stimulating good immune factors like interleukin-2 and gamma interferon which reduces viral loads in hepatitis patients. Nutrient isolation and processing reduces their amounts in plants. Against this backdrop, The Rockefeller Institute of Medical Research warned that, "If the doctor of today do not become the nutritionist of tomorrow, then the nutritionist of today will become the doctor of tomorrow".

The Role of Nutrition in Chronic Inflammations
In inflammatory diseases, the chemical messengers' leukotrines and prostaglandins are manufactured from a type of omega-6 fatty acid called arachidonic acid (AA). When the ratio of omega-3 to omega-6 ratios are balanced one to one, as nature intended, appropriate amounts of omega-6 are produced to respond to inflammatory assault, and healing takes place. But in standard American diets, the ratio of omega-6 far exceeds omega-3 by ratios of 20 to 1. Excess omega-6 generated from malnutrition and acidosis fuels a steady supply of excess arachidonic acid that synthesizes creates an excess of chemical inflammatory messengers. In this situation, the omega-6 fatty acid becomes the friend-turned-foe that has to be stopped. This oversupply of omega-6 fatty acid is the major etiology of chronic inflammatory diseases. It will take about 100 years for the human body to adapt to a 20 : 1 ratio that western diets currently provides (Chilton, 2006).

Modern diets and food production cannot negate human genetics, biochemistry, and physiology laid down millions of years ago. Nature has equipped the human body for ancestral diets; modern food processing creates end products that are totally incompatible with our chemistry. When the Hippocratic Oath which emphasizes "food as medicine" is replaced with "drugs as medicine", degenerative diseases set in. The main cause of the majority of diseases in North America today is malnutrition. In his 1988 Surgeon General's Report, Dr. C. Everett Koop stated "The

American diet is the cause of approximately two-thirds of disease related deaths in America." The American diet will continue to be the culprit as long as we follow a Western "coke, burger and fries" dietary pattern. Chronic degenerative diseases will continue to plague us.

The human body works around the clock, replacing about 300 million dead cells every minute. This replacement is dependent on the spare parts and raw material that are being supplied exogenously. The standard American and Western diets supply the body with dead building blocks which favor the continuation of diseased cells, organs, and organisms (Maklmus and Shockey, 2006). When we replaced millet with processed wheat and consume food devoid of the needed building blocks, the blood borrows from the bones, saliva, and other tissues to sustain the needed pH for survival. This leaves the organs and tissues acidic and oxygen deficient, which sets the stage for degeneration.

Protein Requirements of the Diseased Liver
Vegetable sources of protein are less strenuous to the liver than proteins derived from animal sources, especially red meat. Vegetable sources of protein with their higher proportion of branched-chain amino acids are less burdensome to a sick liver when compared to animal proteins with high levels of aromatic amino acids. It is assumed that most aromatic amino acids are metabolized in the liver while most branched chain amino acids are metabolized in peripheral muscles and hence do not overload the liver.

Nutritionists believe that dietary consumption of proteins must correlate with an individual's body weight. In individuals with liver disease, they recommend approximately 0.9 grams of protein per kilogram (2.2 pounds) of total body weight each day. This translates to about 30 – 100 grams per day or about 25 percent of the daily calories derived from proteins that an individual needs to take. Individuals in good health need about 0.4 g of protein per pound of body weight. For example, an individual weighing 150 pounds will need 0.4 × 150 or 60 g of proteins daily. When going through a disease's stages, more proteins are needed for repair, rebuilding of tissues, and to help fight infection. The intake should be increased to about 0.7 g – 0.8g of protein per pound of body weight. For example, an individual weighing 150 pounds and fighting infection will need about 150×0.7 or 105 g of proteins daily.

What's wrong with Animal Proteins?

When animals are killed, their uric acid remains. Our liver, unlike that of other carnivores, can only eliminate a small amount of the uric acid consumed from meat. Diseased livers cannot tolerate high levels of ammonia, which is a toxic by-product of toxic protein metabolism. When consumed excessively, animal proteins favor the multiplication of unfriendly bacteria over friendly bacteria in the intestine. Ammonia is also formed by the action of proteolytic bacteria in the intestine, which the liver converts it to urea. Diseased livers cannot metabolize urea, which accumulates in the body causing hepatic encephalopathy or mental confusion. Ground beef found in hamburgers, sausages, and hot dogs putrefy easily in the digestive tract. Each meat cell has lysozymes, which are supposed to break down and digest it. When meat is ground, the cells rupture and the enzymes leak out of the cells and self-destruct, which facilitates putrefaction. (Jensen, 1999) Aromatic amino acids from meats products convert easily to ammonia.

- Animal proteins and fatty foods favor the overproduction of male and female hormones, which is a catalyst for cancer development.
- When we cook meat products, we destroy all the nutrients and enzymes.
- Meat protein supplies more than the daily protein requirement of the body (Malkmus and Shockey, 2006)

Branched chain amino acids are beneficial in the management of nitrogen balance in the liver. Non-meat protein sources like soy, legumes, whole grains, and vegetables are good sources of proteins that help keep ammonia levels under control in cirrhotic patients.

Doctor's health advisory: If you must consume meat, eat free-range poultry and fowl grown without hormones, and sea foods caught in the wild as opposed to farm-raised sea foods. If you crave red meat, reserve it for Sunday brunch please.

Carbohydrates Requirements of the Liver

Carbohydrates are starches that are metabolized to sugars for the energy needs of cells. They are the fuel source for the body .They are broken down into glucose and glycogen by the liver when energy is needed. Complex carbohydrates are preferred over simple carbohydrates in the management of liver patients because they provide energy levels that are sustained over longer periods of time. Hepatitis challenges the ability of the liver to regulate blood glucose levels. Unlike simple sugars, complex carbohydrates do not cause the blood sugar fluctuations associated with simple sugars.

Simple carbohydrates and refined sugars are metabolized to fat and triglycerides by the liver, which becomes burdensome to the diseased liver. They clog arteries and hamper organ functions, and can build up in the liver where they contribute to fatty liver. They are also deposited in other body organs. . Simple carbohydrates turn on fat production in cells and turn off fat-burning cells in the body, causing organ degeneration and weight gain.

Nutritionists recommend that individuals with liver disease should opt for a diet that supplies about 60 percent of the complex carbohydrates, which should translate into about 400 grams of carbohydrates daily. If diet is not providing this amount, the liver will derive its energy from proteins and fats which leads to muscle-wasting diseases. This also happens if there is too much protein and not enough carbohydrates *"Sugar is the most hazardous foodstuff in the American diet" Dr Linus Pauling* to meets the liver's daily need. This constitutes an added strain on an already diseased liver because converting protein to energy is more taxing than converting carbohydrates to energy. Consuming too much fat and not enough carbohydrates (e.g. too much salad dressings) will exacerbate fatty liver disease.

Can I use White Sugar?

Manufacture of white sugar starts with synthetic chemicals and charcoal. Raw sugar is a complex carbohydrate that contains all the synergistic properties of whole foods. Refined sugar, a simple carbohydrate, is a fractioned, artificial, and devitalized by-product of the original compound. The end product is refeeed to as sucrose-a crystallized acid. It encourages the proliferation of unfriendly bacteria and viruses in the digestive tract. In the metabolism of refined sugar, the body has to borrow from its own reserve of nutrients. (Dufty, 1993).

Natural fructose is commonly processed into high fructose. In their 2005 book, *Beating Cancer with Nutrition*, authors Patrick and Noreen Quillin indicate that Americans consume 15 billion gallons of soft drinks, 2.7 billion donuts, and 500 million Twinkies™ per year. They indicate that our appetite for sugar parallels the astronomical increase in the increase of chronic degenerative diseases. It has found its way into products like Equal™, Splenda™, Sweet and Low™, Coca-Cola™, all soft drinks, wines, alcoholic beverages, fruit juices, sweeteners, cookies, pies, candies, cakes, ice creams, jams, jellies, desserts, ketchup, confections, children's vitamins, and tobacco products.

Sugar and white flour suppresses the immune system by making the white blood cells dormant, drugged, clumped together, mutate out of control, pre-cancerous, and sluggish (Malkmus and Shockey 2006).

Today the average person consumes about 170 pounds of sugar per year which translates into about 50 teaspoons of sugar per day. A 12-ounce can of soda contains about 11 teaspoons of sugar. The average person consumes two or three sodas daily which translates into about 22 – 33 tablespoons of sugar daily. This dietary habit puts the immune system on hold while diseases and pathogens take a strong hold on the body (Malkmus and Shockey 2006).

Most sugar alternatives like NutraSweet™ and Equal™ contain aspartame, a triple molecule composed of aspartic acid (a neurotoxin), phenylalanine, and methyl alcohol (wood alcohol). Methyl alcohol is converted to formaldehyde, a neurotoxin in the body. "A partial list of products containing aspartame [includes] diet soft drinks, breakfast cereals, malt beverages, pie filings, tea, fruit juice concentrates, baked goods, frostings, breath mints, chewing gum, wine coolers, yogurt, [and] chewable multivitamins. It is used as [a flavoring] in Mylanta™, Centrum™ vitamins, and children's Tylenol™ (O'Shea, 2004, pp31-33).

Doctor's health advisory: The best dietary sources of sugars are raw unrefined honey, raw unrefined sugar cane, or fruits. The best dietary sources of complex carbohydrates are pasta, beans, whole grain breads, and brown rice.

Fat Requirements of the Liver
Fats are the body's reservoir of excess energy. They are very concentrated sources of calories. They are used as energy sources in extreme situations. They supply more calories than most of the other nutrients we consume. Excessive consumption of fatty foods can result in weight gain and fatty liver disease. Individuals can have fatty livers and still not be overweight.

Animal proteins, especially farm-raised and domesticated animals, have more saturated fat contents than those that roam freely in the wild. Saturated fats in animals are store houses for toxins, and when we consume animals we have to deals with these toxins.

How much fat can I take?
The following formula should help you determine you caloric goal:
- If you are underweight, multiply your body weight in pounds by 18 to give your caloric goal.
- If you have normal weight, multiply your body weight in pounds by 16 to give your caloric goal.
- If you are overweight, multiply your body weight in pounds by 14 to give you your caloric goal.

Fat should never exceed about 20 percent of your daily dietary intake. Fat are needed for the absorption of the fat-soluble vitamins A, D, E and K, which are deficient in people with cholestatic liver diseases. Fats help foods taste better, especially in cirrhotic patients who don't have much appetite.

Essential fatty acids. In 1937, Dr. Szent-Gyorgyi was awarded the Nobel Prize for discovering that essential fatty acids enhance cellular oxygenation when combined with sulphur-rich proteins. They are a must have for individuals with liver diseases. They are healing fats needed for efficient functioning of the liver and bodily functions. Essential fatty acids are major components of cell membranes. They are precursors to molecules such as prostaglandins and other antioxidants that assist liver detoxification. They give us healthy life rather than the shelf life we get from hydrogenated oils. Their deficiencies compromise cellular integrity, make the cell membranes porous, and jeopardize the ability of cells to eliminate toxins (Cabot,

1996). Omega-3 fatty acids have been shown to inhibit aggressive forms of liver cancers (Arthur, 2006). The omega-3 fatty acids are one of the essential fatty acids and nutrients that the body cannot manufacture. They have to be ingested directly from food or food supplements. They are required for optimal cellular functioning, cellular communications, and reversal of degenerative diseases, structural cellular integrity, cellular respiration, and overall health.

Dietary sources of EFAs includes flax seeds, hemp seeds, soy beans, walnuts, pumpkin seeds, dark green vegetables, cold-water fish, and marine animals. A dosage of 200 mg – 2 grams daily is ideal.

Doctor's health advisory: Never use essential fatty acids for cooking. They should not be exposed to excessive sunlight as they may turn rancid. Delight yourself with three to four tablespoons of cold-pressed organic EFAs daily. Always refrigerate EFAs, and never buy EFAs from a health food store if they are not in a refrigerator. Like coconut oil, EFAs do not raise your cholesterol.

Chapter 6

A Supplemental Approach to Healing Liver Disease

Healing the liver with vitamins, suppliments and antioxidants

Before embarking on any conventional remedy, it is best to ask the doctor on what lifestyle changes you should embark, like eating habits and exercise programs. Always have it in your mind that drugs will never cure your condition. They will treat the symptoms while nature works on the immune system to heal you from within. Even though your doctor may not agree with this, it is true. Delay drugs and embark on aggressive lifestyle changes unless your situation is in an emergency, interventional, or critical stage. Ask your doctor what the cause of your illness is. If your doctor doesn't know the cause of your illness, search the Internet. Ask other doctors or alternative care providers about the possible causes of your illness. When you have some answers, take the results to your doctor, and start working on the solution from the causes. These views are congruent with that of Dr. Gloria Gilbere who said *"Knowledge of the cause is power over the disease."* Dr. Gilbere overcame fibromyalgia, leaky-gut syndrome, and multiple chemical sensitivities with the knowledge of alternative remedies after she had tried conventional approaches without much success. *We believe if you don't know what's wrong, you can't make it right.*

Of all human desires, food is the first and the greatest, because newborns cry for food immediately after they are born. The sex drive does not develop until the time of puberty. This desire for food remains dominant until we die (Bronner Jr., 2000). While nutritionists believe that by correcting malnutrition we can rectify the majority of diseases, I believe lifestyle, cultural factors, emotional states, belief systems, religion, and psychological factors drive dietary patterns. The depth of our attitudes about food drives the strength of our aptitudes and appetites for food.

Attitudinal healing is crucial because our dietary patterns are influenced by our belief systems, religious affiliations, social factors, environmental factors, cultural biases, emotional states, and peer pressures. Studies show that 85 percent of the causes of illnesses that afflict man are psychosomatic in origin, 5 percent are genetic, and only 10 percent are due to physical factors that require drugs and herbal remedies as mentioned earlier in this book. While medicine blames our genes for our diseases, the majority of the illnesses we suffer today were either non-existent of there were fewer than 3 percent of such degenerative diseases in the early 1900's. This implies that our forefathers did not pass them down to us. Studies that show that identical or fraternal twins raised under different environments responded differently to the same medicine were corroborated by the writings of Nobel Laureate Barbara Mcclintock who concluded that our lifestyle and environment play a much more overwhelming role in influencing our state of health than our genes. Our environments, diet, and thought patterns shape our biography that ultimately determines our biology. Our biology becomes our biochemistry.

This implies that all the herbs, nutrient vitamins, hospitalizations, and drugs we use to fight diseases are only addressing about 10 percent of what is needed to influence healing. While mainstream medicine has aimed to treat physical symptoms without looking at the spiritual component, it has always failed to restore wholeness because separating the mind from the body is like separating currents from electricity or waves from the ocean. Healing words must compliment herbs to attain optimum health, i.e. minding the body while mending the mind.

Herbal remedies are definitely not as dramatic as drugs when used under professional supervision. They elicit fewer side effects. But, like drugs, they block some enzymatic reactions to elicit therapeutic effects and some do have adverse reactions like other pharmaceutical agents. (Strand, 2003). Like drugs, when we take combination of herbal remedies that utilize the same enzyme systems, bottle necks and back ups are created. This is what is responsible for some of the hypersensitivity or allergic reactions associated with herbs. This is to be expected when drugs and herbs utilize the same enzyme systems.

Since conventional medicine has not been able to effectively heal anybody from degenerative liver diseases, it serves the general public for the government to invest adequate resources to establish the safety and efficacy of complimentary alternative remedies, e.g. like regulatory agencies such as the FDA to monitor their use. The medical community has consistently paid little attention to the use of herbal remedies while putting undue focus of their toxicity. This has not stopped the increased use of alternatives because conventional remedies in the management of infective hepatitis and other chronic degenerative diseases have up until now been fraught with disappointing results. Most of the information on herbs are gathered by the word of mouth or through anecdotal evidence because herb manufacturers do not have the kind of resources and promotional know-how employed by pharmaceutical companies to study their safety and efficacy. Germany, Japan, and China have allowed extensive studies of herbal remedies to be done and have incorporated their use into mainstream health care. This has not occurred in the United States because of intense lobbying by the pharmaceutical industry and the American Medical Association that feel threatened by the use of alternative remedies. Currently, there are no quality control measures in the manufacture of herbs. Hence, there are no guarantees that capsules and tablets contain what is advertised on their container labels. There are no organizations or governmental agency to protect the consumers. There have been documented cases of herbal remedies that do not contain the advertised active ingredients or have too much of the ingredients advertised.

Each individual has a unique constitution that favors the right mix of nutrients. We differ in the quantities of nutrients we each need to attain health. One man's remedy can be another man's poison. An excellent liver remedy for your auntie might be your nightmare. We differ in food preferences which are reflected in our biochemical and physiological differences. We need to pay attention to how different remedies, herbs, and nutrients impart and affect our energy levels, moods, and body. It takes a determined effort and a willing heart to change established mental and physical factors that have made us ill. If we are not cognizant of the physiological signal generated within our bodies regarding illness, we begin a process that removes our awareness from our own nature. We end up making poor lifestyle choices that gradually result in physical degeneration. What is good for us depends more on what our body needs than expert opinion. It took a long time for negative factors to make our bodies susceptible to disease, so it will take diligence and patience for our internal environments to defy illness (Erasmus, 1993).

Selenium

Several studies have shown that low levels and depletion of selenium in hepatitis B and C patients tend to correlate with progression of disease severity. Studies also show that hepatitis B and C patients have significantly lower levels of zinc and glutathione and high levels of oxidative stress. Once selenium has been used up in the host infected cells, hepatitis B and C viruses infect adjacent cells.

Selenium is a trace mineral the body uses to produce glutathione peroxidase, which is part of the body's antioxidant defense systems. Glutathione peroxidase uses selenium to break down rancid fats without releasing free radicals. Selenium works with vitamin E to protect cell membranes from free radical damages and increases glutathione activities. Even though it is a trace mineral, it is only required in minute amounts. Selenium supplements offer protection against certain types of cancers. Plants are the major sources of selenium but its contents in animals or plants depend on the soil where the animals or plants are grown. Animals that eat grains or plants grown in selenium-rich soil have higher levels of selenium. Its depletion corresponds to the severity of liver diseases in general. It enhances lymphocyte proliferation and increases antibodies. *Selenium is found mostly in garlic, legumes, cereals, and whole grains grown in selenium-rich soil. These include oats, whole wheat bread, Brazil nuts, red Swiss chard, brown rice, mushrooms, broccoli, onions, brewers yeast, turnips, orange juice, and barley. It is also found in animal products like meats and sea foods. The recommended dose is 100 mg per day. It is usually toxic in doses above 250 mg. Because most of the food grown in the United States is deficient in selenium, I highly recommend supplementation.*

Doctors Health advisory: Herbalists have used a combination of medicinal mushrooms, selenium, and olive leaf extract with great success in combatting hepatitis B, hepatitis C, and the HIV virus.

Folic acid: Folic acid, a crucial member of the B vitamins, is used by the liver to enhance healthy methylation that is an essential component of enzymatic detoxification in the liver. Deficiency of folic acid is associated with high levels of lipoperoxidases which is an indicator of ongoing free radical damage in the liver.

Vitamins (Co-Enzymes). For enzymes to bring about change, they need helpers or igniters. These helpers are called co-enzymes which are referred to as vitamins. The co-enzymes ignite amino acids building blocks from food into biologically active proteins which the body uses to manufacture almost everything from infection-fighting white bloods cells to muscles. The enzymes and the co-enzymes orchestrate ultra-sophisticated biological activities called a "complex." The enzyme complex is what leads to enzymatic activities. When these co-enzymes are deficient, the complex cannot be formed, and deficiency disease occurs. Vitamins are essential in small quantities for normal functioning of the body. Enzymes cannot work without these co-factors and minerals. Cooperation, synergy, and co-factoring are needed for enzymatic activity to occur.

Enzymes are the organic catalyst that increases the speed of biochemical reactions in the body. In plant life, enzymes make seeds sprout, fruits ripen, leaves change color, and a wide variety of biochemical activities. If enzymes are absent, reactions could not take place at the normal body temperatures of 98.4°F (Yiamouyiannis, 1986). Enzymes are the agents responsible for change. They are a group of synthesized amino acids that change other substances to a form that is usable by liver cells. The enzyme systems in the liver are called microsomal enzyme systems. Every chemical change that takes place in the liver is mediated by the activities of enzymes. The life functions of cells are mediated by the actions of enzymes just like an automobile needs the ignition. Enzymes are long chain amino acids held in specific shapes by hydrogen bonds. These shapes have to match the corresponding co-enzyme (vitamin) like a lock and key.

In 1905, Englishman William Fletcher determined that if special factors are absent from foods, diseases ensures. He discovered that the disease beriberi was caused by eating processed (polished) rice. He was of the opinion that there were special nutrients in the husks of the rice. In 1906, English biochemist Sir Frederic Gowland Hopkins discovered that certain food factors were important to health and, if deficient, diseases occurred. In 1912, Polish Scientist Casmir Funk named these deficient factors vitamins. Together, Hopkins and Funk formulated the vitamin hypothesis of deficiency diseases.

Beta-carotene is converted to vitamin A in the body. Vitamin A exhibits anti-cancer properties with people who have cirrhosis. It helps to prevent the progression of liver cirrhosis to hepatocellular carcinoma. As co-enzymes, it facilitates the synthesis of antibodies like T cells and other natural killer cells.

Doctor's health advisory: Dietary sources of beta carotene are carrots, peaches, apricots, sweet potato, beets, tomatoes, kale, squash, green pears, collards, cantaloupe, cayenne pepper, hot peppers, and broccoli.

The B vitamins are water soluble and are not stored in the body. Excessive amounts are flushed out of the body. This necessitates the need to replenish the body with these vitamins daily from food sources. Mental, physical, and oxidative stress, alcohol, tobacco, caffeine, excessive sugar, food preservatives, drugs, and environmental toxins deplete the levels of B vitamins in the body. The B vitamins include vitamins B1 thiamine, B2 riboflavin, B3 niacin, B5 pantothenic acid, B6 pyridoxine, and B12 cyanocobalamin. Vitamin B12 is necessary for rebuilding new liver cells, as it needed for the metabolism of fats and proteins in liver cells. It works synergistically with vitamin B6. Vitamin B6 facilitates the absorption of Vitamin B12.

Fat-soluble vitamins require not only adequate dietary intake but also good digestion and assimilation by the body. Normal bile production is essential for the metabolism of these vitamins. If bile production is poor, oral supplementation of the fat-soluble vitamins may not be enough to restore them to normal in patients with degenerative liver disease.

Vitamin C is a potent anti-oxidant that works synergistically with vitamin E to arrest oxidative liver damage. Vitamin E oil protects lipid membranes from oxidative damage and corrects deficiencies caused by mal-absorption of fats and oils. Mervyn (1983) attributes liver cirrhosis, obstructive jaundice, and pancreatic insufficiency as conditions that arise from mal-absorption of fats and oils. Vitamin C and E can block the formation of nitrosamines which can prevent the activation of the P450 enzyme systems, and retard tumor proliferation and formation. The liver cells incorporate vitamin E into lipoproteins which then transport it to various tissues in the body. Vitamin E helps reduce the ability of the stellate cells to manufacture scar cirrhotic tissues. This ultimately hampers the scar tissue formation. The E vitamins from vegetable juice soften and loosen the formed scars which ultimately allow for easier passage of blood through the liver. This reduces backups in the spleen, pancreas, and ascites, and facilitates the supply of essential nutrients to the liver, hence its role in the regeneration of the liver cells. The E vitamins similarly aid in the maintenance of high levels of glutathione which are reduced during hepatitis inflammation.

Foods that contain the C vitamins are rose hips, kale, parsley, collard greens, mustard greens, cauliflower, red cabbage, strawberries, papaya, spinach, kiwi fruit, citrus fruits, asparagus, mangos, oranges, peppers, broccoli, and Brussels sprouts. The B vitamins are found in cruciferous vegetables, brewers yeast, bee pollen, green leafy vegetables, and fruit. Foods that contain vitamin E include almonds and sunflower seeds, avocados, asparagus, walnuts, tomatoes, whole grains, nuts, wheat germ, and green leafy vegetables.

Vitamin K greatly helps to lower the deficiency of clotting factors that are deficient during inflammatory liver disease. People with cirrhosis bruise easily due to vitamin K deficiency. The liver uses this co-enzyme to make prothrombin which is needed for blood clotting. Bacteria in the intestines manufactures vitamin K. *Dietary sources of vitamin K are green leafy vegetables, whole grains, cabbage and organ meats.*

Vitamins and the Anti-oxidation Systems
Vitamins are very critical components of the anti-oxidation system. The anti-oxidation system is second only to the microsomal liver detoxification system. The anti-oxidation process is similar to what goes on when iron rusts, when apple exposed to air turns brown, or when butter becomes rancid. In a balanced healthy state, the rate of formation of free radicals is always balanced by the rate of consumption of antioxidants. When the balance between free-radical generation and anti-oxidant defense is unfavorable, oxidative damage and degenerative disease begins.

Anti-oxidants work by scavenging excess free radicals and neutralizing them. Diets of whole organic and unprocessed foods, vegetables, and fruit juices are the best sources of anti-oxidants. There are two types of anti-oxidants defenses—chemical and biochemical. Chemical antioxidants are scavengers of free radicals that stabilize them by giving them electrons they needed to be neutralized. These are found mainly in vitamins A, E, C, beta-carotene, glutathione, bioflavonoid, selenium, zinc, Co-enzyme Q10, and green tea. Biochemical anti-oxidants scavenge free radicals and prevent their regeneration. They include lipoid acid, superoxide dismutase (SOD), and a wide variety of repair enzymes (Byrnes, 2005; Baker, 2004; and Bland and Benum, 1999)

Vitamin C, E, B12, bioflavinoids, beta-carotene, glutathione, selenium, and zinc work synergistically as antioxidants during free-radical attacks as follows. A vitamin C molecule gives the "victimized" molecule that encounters free radical damage a replacement electron. Vitamin C then receives a replacement electron from a molecule of the bioflavonoid. Next, the bioflavonoid molecule receives a replacement electron from a beta carotene molecule. The beta-carotene molecule, in turn, receives a replacement electron from a vitamin E molecule. Finally, the vitamin E molecule receives a replacement electron from glutathione. Any of these anti-oxidants cannot work alone, and deficiency of any of the antioxidants in the above mix will lead to free-radical damage. If one antioxidant is missing in the process, the anti-oxidation stops and oxidative damage begins (Baker, 2004).

Doctors Health advisory: No amount of vitamins, minerals, or herbal remedies can fix an upset mind, a broken spirit, and an unforgiving spirit.

What is Hypervitaminosis?

Unsupervised and excessive use of vitamins creates a condition referred to as hypervitaminosis or vitamin toxicity. Often times, theses reactions can cause tremendous damage to the liver and negate the initial treatment goal. In the management of liver diseases, only minute quantities of vitamins and minerals derived from food sources are needed for complex biochemical reactions in the body. The aim of

"The right mix of nutrients will eradicate most diseases."
Dr. Linus Pauling

treatment should be getting just the right mix of nutrients in the most synergistic and balanced form to jumpstart immuno-compromised individuals. Synergy is best obtained when the right foods are eaten in the right combination at much lower doses than supplementation. Nutrient supplementation with pills bypasses the body's own innate ability to draw nutrients from food. This makes the digestive system atrophy and lazy if it gets used to pre-absorbed foods in pill forms. The innate ability to selectively absorb and excrete nutrients from whole food is lost with isolated supplements (Colbin, 1998). The isolation and manufacture of multivitamins requires the use of a number of processes, especially the use of heat to extract the vitamins. The application of heat during processing destroys the enzymatic catalyst that the body needs for cellular regeneration. Research shows that high levels of isolated vitamin supplements overwhelm immuno-compromised livers and exacerbates biochemical imbalances that cause degenerative diseases.

Whole foods are too complex for simple chemical classification of synthetic isolated supplements. Isolated supplements have properties different from their parent sources, the totality of which is greater than the sum of isolated parts (Mowrey, 1986). Whole food are complex structures made from organic transformations which involve the natural conversions of inorganic nutrients in the soil into organic, ionized foods, potentiated by probiotic microorganisms and enzymes (Rubin, 2006). Most natural vitamin supplements are usually more than 90 percent synthetic and they have neither integrity nor food value. Synthetic vitamin supplements are sometimes better at reducing excess than supplementing deficiencies. They confuse the liver in its metabolic role. Long-term supplementation with isolated vitamins neither cures or prevents serious diseases (Pitchford, 2002)

Since the FDA does not require manufacturers of supplements to test their products for safety and purity, most multivitamin formulas are synthetic, petroleum-derived vitamins made with industrial-grade mineral salts. Microscopically, isolated vitamins have a crystalline appearance while food nutrients have a rounded and smaller appearance. Scientists believe that smaller particle size improves bioavailability and absorption. Bioavailability is best obtained from whole foods. Isolated USP vitamins are analogues to natural ingredients which have no vitamin activity. They act as a vitamin antagonist or produce deficiency symptoms of the specific vitamins for which they are analogues (Thiel, 2004). The mythical consequence of the chemical extraction and isolation of nutrients from whole plants is that "it kills the intelligence of the plant and when a remedy is devoid of its intelligence, it becomes lifeless and of no use to disease management" (Sharma, Mishra and Meade, 2002).

The UL is the index set by the National Academies of Science for the maximum daily intake of a nutrient that is likely to pose no risk or adverse effects in healthy people. Centrum™ Performance Complete Multivitamins, Twin Lab™ Men's Ultra, and Puritan's Pride™ Mega Vita Gel Softgels exceed the UL for the vitamin B niacin. Excessive amount of niacin (above 35mg per day) in the above supplements can cause liver damage in unsupervised clinical settings. One in four supplements sold to consumers either exceeds or contains less that the amount of active ingredients listed on its label. These supplements contain herbicides, insecticides, and heavy metals like lead or arsenic. Consequently, they do not disintegrate properly and are not properly absorbed in the body (Cooperman, 2006).

Particle size and physiochemical form of nutrients play a major role in the bioavailability of nutrients and vitamins to the body. From a biochemical point of view, chemically derived vitamins are structurally and molecularly similar to that found in whole foods but bio-energenetically different. Energetic patterns of chemically-derived molecules are flat and harshly geometric, while vegetable-derived molecules have vibrant, variable, and artistic molecular geometry (Thiel, 2004). The bio-energetic patterns are the living energies in herbs that facilitate their bioavailability and subsequent absorption by the liver (Tips, 2002).

Ascorbic Acid versus Vitamin C?
Ascorbic acid is often isolated from the vitamin C complex. Ascorbic acid is the commercially-available form of vitamin C. The vitamin C complex in fruits and vegetables consists of ascorbic acid, flavonoids, polyphenols, catechins, rutins, enzymes, and thousands of unknown alkaloids. Ascorbic acid is only a small part of the whole complex (the outer shell of the enzyme). The isolation of ascorbic acid from whole food eliminates the anti-oxidant's synergistic actions of the complex, making it incompatible with the biochemistry of human organ systems.

Beta-Carotene versus Vitamin A
Beta-carotene is biochemically and bio-energetically different from vitamin A. Unsupervised use of vitamin A supplements, which are metabolized to retinoid, is associated with hepatoxicity, tetratogenicity, and carcinogenicity. Conversely, when carotenoids are ingested in large amounts, their anti-oxidant properties neutralize the free-radical damage of the retinoid in the complex-a synergistic process. While excess vitamin A is toxic to the body, excess beta-carotene is non-toxic and excreted through the kidneys.

Natural versus Synthetic Vitamin E

The term "natural" is often misleading when dealing with vitamins. Manufacturers of vitamin supplements can have only about 10 percent of the natural supplement and 90 percent of the synthetic prototype and still label their products "natural". So buyers beware! Read the labels, or you may be sacrificing quality for price with the choices you make.

Alpha tocopherol is the scientific name of the vitamin E used by the body. There are other varieties that synergistically work with alpha tocopherol, namely beta tocopherol, gamma tocopherol, and delta tocopherol, which are all collectively referred to as mixed tocopherol. The mixed tocopherols have been shown to increase the effectiveness and bioavailability of the vitamin E activity of D alpha tocopherol. Isolating any one component of these from food totally negates their synergistic ability to influence healing as the whole is always greater than the sum of the individual parts. Biochemically, vitamin E is either right handed or left handed, often referred to as the D form and the L form. Scientists believe that the more bioavailable of the two and the most often used by the body is the D form, referred to as D-alpha tocopherol. Scientists have not yet to discover the function of the L form in the body. When vitamin E is made synthetically, the D and L forms are often bound together to form an entirely new compound called DL-alpha tocopherol which the body does not recognize. The bioactive D-alpha tocopherol is not available to the tissues.

Food sources of vitamin E are avocados, kiwi, nectarines, grapes, peaches, beet roots, animal livers, and adrenals.

Co-enzyme Q10: Co-enzyme Q10 is a compound that exists naturally in the energy-producing centers of cells called mitochondria. It is responsible from the manufacture of ATP, the energy source of cells. It also helps the body utilize oxygen more efficiently, thus combating fatigue and helps to stave off cancer in liver patients. ATP fuels significant numbers of biochemical reactions and protein synthesis. Co-enzyme Q10 is an antioxidant that protects liver cells from the consequences of reduced blood flow or ischemia. It protects the cellular mitochondria and cell membranes from oxidative damage. Co-enzyme Q10 helps stimulate the immune system, leading to higher numbers and levels of the T-cells and macrophages. Since it dissolves readily in fat, it enforces its anti-oxidant activity in the cell membranes. *Dietary sources of co-enzyme Q10 are oily fish and organ meats like liver. Vegetable sources of Co-enzyme Q10 are unprocessed spinach, broccoli, peanuts, wheat germ, and whole grains. A dosage of 30 – 200 mg daily is recommended.*

Doctors Health Advisory: A dosage 150 – 250 mg daily is ideal for a liver patient. See the list of products in the appendix.

Alpha Lipoic Acid: Alpha lipoic acid is a fat-soluble anti-oxidant and anti-cancer agent that can penetrate cell membranes to exert their therapeutic actions. Since it is both water and lipid soluble, it exerts its anti-oxidant activities on lipid-soluble cell membranes and water soluble membranes. It helps rid the body and the liver of heavy metals that hamper organ functions. As a scavenger, it helps chelate heavy metals. It enhance the activity of glutathione, and reduces the level of hepatic fibrosis associated with liver injury. *Dietary sources of alpha lipoic acid include spinach, broccoli, beef, brewers yeast, and organ meats like kidney and the heart. A dosage of 30 – 200 mg daily is ideal.*

Potassium: Often given as injection or as potassium chloride, it helps alleviate abdominal and leg swelling in individuals with complications of cirrhosis. While sodium retains water potassium help dispel excess fluids from the body by shifting the osmotic balance. Potassium chloride is often used like table salt to season food. Potassium chloride

Doctor's health advisory: Potassium is contraindicated in individuals with kidney problems and in people taking potassium.

Zinc: Zinc inhibits replication of diverse viruses in vitro. Zinc deficiency is common in cirrhosis. It helps activate the enzyme glutamine synthetase. Zinc helps bind and remove copper from the body and is used in management of patients with Wilson disease. Zinc deficiency reduces T-lymphocyte numbers and decreases immunological responses to diseases. Zinc stimulates the production and action of the thymic hormones and regulates T-cell maturation. Along with selenium, it helps sustain blood levels of glutathione.

SAMe: S-adenosylmethionine (SAMe) discovered in 1952 in Italy is synthesized from the combination of amino acid L-methionine, folic acid, vitamin B12, and trimethylglycine. SAMe is a methylation agent that facilitates the synthesis of glutathione. SAMe decreases the production of liver collagen which leads to the formation of fibrous tissues. SAMe is necessary in the synthesis of all sulphur-containing compounds. It facilitates bile flow and relieves cholestasis. Low amounts of folate (B9) in the body may lead to decreased levels of sAMe. SAMe is not found in food, so it has to be supplemented directly from exogenous sources. If sAMe levels are depleted, the liver's ability to manufacture bile, amino acids, or eliminate methionene, whose level can be toxic, is hampered. SAMe regulates the content of fats and fluids in the body and deters the formation of fatty levers. Lipotropic agents like choline, betaine, methionine, vitamin B6, folic acid, and vitamin B12 facilitate the flow of bile and fat to and from the liver and increase the levels of sAMe and glutathione. Dietary sources of methionine and cysteine are red peppers, garlic, onions, broccoli, Brussel sprouts, sesame seeds, whole grains, barley, sirloin, chickpeas, lentils, cottage cheese, eggs, oat meal, and wheat.

Aloe Vera: The healing juice
One of the most versatile herbs that enhance the activities of macrophages is aloe vera. There are more than 250 known biologically active nutrients and alkaloids in aloe vera and thousands of yet to be discovered phytonutrients. They include vitamins, minerals, prostangladins, essential fatty acids, anthraquinones, and mucopolysaccarises. The mucopolysaccarides establish themselves in the cell membranes of the liver cells and body cells, fortify the cell wall, and make the cells more resistant to pathogens and viruses. The mucopolysaccarides (Acemannan) exhibit antiviral, anti-inflammatory, and immune-stimulating characteristics by optimizing cellular metabolism. The receptor sites of the immune cells (macrophages) and one of the sugars of aloe vera polysaccharides called D-mannos have a lock-and-key relationship, i.e. they have a bio-synergistic fit (Quillin and Quillin, 2005). This bio-synergistic fit is what makes aloe vera elicit its healing properties in the body. Heating and processing disrupts this aloe function. In his book, *Triumph over Hepatitis C*, Lloyd Wright, a chronic hepatitis sufferer, chronicles the following characteristics of aloe vera:

- It enhances macrophage activities, making them more phagocytic; it engulfs foreign matter.
- It enhances the ability of macrophages to modulate the immune system.

- It enhances macrophages' ability to stimulate and regulate the production and release of antibodies and the needed interferons required for immune functions.
- It increases the activities of the T lymphocytes which are important regulators and co-coordinators of the immune system.
- It assists with cellular detoxification, relieves arthritic pain associated with hepatitis, and stimulates bone marrow functions.

Doctors Health advisory: I strongly recommend fresh organic aloe vera from a health food store to make juices from them. Read the label and make sure you buy 100 percent organic, preservative-free, unheated and unprocessed aloe vera. Heating and processing destroys the polysaccharides, its active ingredient.

Online Resources for Dietary Supplements
- The National Institutes of Health Office of Dietary Supplements: http://ods.od.nih.gov/index.aspx
- International bibliographic information on dietary supplements http://grande.nal.usda.gov/ibids/index.php
- http://www.healthfreedom.info/index.htm
- http://www.oxfordjournals.org/

What is Interferon?
Interferons were discovered in 1954 by Dr. Yasuhiko Kojima, while working with an associate, Yasuichi Nagano. Interferons and interleukins are a family of chemical substances called cytokines. They are secreted by the activated helper T cells in response to antigens. As a collection of proteins and chemical mediators, they are released by the body and tissue cells in injured areas during inflammation against viral infection and cancer.

Our cells build several different types of interferon—alpha, beta and omega. The largest groups are about 20 types of alpha interferon made by nearly all cells. They are used to mobilize our first line of non-specific defense mechanisms against invading organisms before the immune system has a chance to get started. They function as immune stimulants and regulators, and are responsible for communication between cells.

The alpha inteferons are produced by the actions of T-cells and macrophages. During viral infection, they stimulate natural killer cells to kill "virus-infected host cells." The gamma inteferons, made by infected T–lymphocytes and natural killer cells, that are sensitive to foreign antigens present in the body, send messages to other cells of the immune systems telling them to focus on cell-based defenses. They also activate the macrophages and arm them with nitric oxide to help clean up the residual mess.

The interferon mechanism is like 'biological martyrdom'- the suffering of death on account of adherence to a cause .Some cells that become causalities of a particular disease choose to, or are programmed to die so as to prevent the spread of the disease to other body parts. This intelligent and innate process cannot be artificially produced in capsules. Intelligence is not synthetic. It is like man playing God. We propose creating an enabling environment for this process to occur naturally. As we supply the body with needed nutrients and make necessary lifestyle changes, the interferon levels of the body is restored, alkalinity is attained, oxidation replaces fermentation and healing takes place

What Does Interferon Do During An Attack?
The activity of interferons is like a system that makes a rotten apple in a basket self-destruct itself before contaminating the whole basket. Similarly, interferons makes virus-infected host cells self-destruct to prevent infecting the whole organism. Failure of the interferon system is assumed to be responsible for the infectiveness of viral infections and cellular degenerative diseases.

When a cell has been attacked, it signals unaffected neighboring cells to produce certain proteins to protect themselves and to localize the infection while concurrently activating other arms of the immune system to call the natural killer cells and macrophages into action. When a host cell gets a target (e.g. virus) from the interferons, it builds specialized proteins to fight the infection (e.g. infected host cells construct enzymes that degrade the RNA or protein synthesis of viral proteins). Consequently, these host cells also chop up their own messenger RNA and "interfere" with their normal protein synthesis or life cycle. The implication of this is that interferon forces infected human cells to self-destruct and shorten their lifespan. .This ultimately slows a growth to crawl.

How Do I Produce Interferons Naturally?
Try Probiotics

The digestive tract is home to more than 100 trillion bacteria of more than 400 species of the good and bad bugs that are supposed to co-exist to maintain a balance about 85 percent

"Champions keep playing until they get it right."
Billie Jean King

friendly bacteria and about 15 percent bad guys. Probiotic literally means pro-life, for life, and life-supporting or friendly. These are microorganisms that sustain the ecological systems of the digestive tract. Probiotics contrast with antibiotic which are anti-life. While probiotics supports and sustains the integrity of beneficial bacteria in the gut, antibiotics indiscriminately destroy the good and the bad bugs in the intestinal tract and creates an imbalance. An efficient lymphatic system is necessary for an efficient immune system. Over 75 percent of the lymphatic system is located in the gut and its tissues are referred to as the gut-associated lymphoid tissue (GALT). To sustain the integrity of the lymphatic system, we must use probiotics along with lifestyle changes to maintain our digestive health.

In the early 1900's, Dr. Metchnikoff, a Nobel Prize winning Russian biologist discovered the presence of probiotics in the digestive tract where they acidify the gut. He proposed that these acid-producing organisms in fermented diary products help sustain friendly bacteria in the gut and prevented fouling in the large intestine. These acid-producing flora protect the gut from overgrowth of competing microorganisms, and the acid they produce makes the digestive tract hostile to disease causing bacteria. In this health state, the populations of harmful bacteria are balanced by the competing good bacteria because of a mutually-interdependent relationship among them. This condition restores proper bacteria ratio and is referred to as *symbiosis*. Since the bacteria in the intestine are busy competing with each other, they do not have time left to cause infections and harm to the digestive system. By lowering the population of harmful bacteria, probiotics displace and consume hardened wastes in the intestines, create conducive environments for beneficial bacteria which act as immune regulators to prep the walls of the intestine for proper absorption of nutrients.

The friendly bacteria also help in the manufacture of some A, B, and K vitamins. These probiotic bacteria also produce substances called bacteriocins which are natural antibiotics that suppress the population of unfriendly bacteria. They produce specialized acids that hinder the colonization of the harmful bacteria, make the gut environment unfriendly to disease-causing pathogens, and acidify the intestinal tract, thus hindering fouling in the large intestine. In situations where the populations of the bad bugs outnumber the good bugs, the imbalance dysbiosis occurs. Scientists believe intestinal dysbyosis is the etiology of all diseases that plague mankind.

Conditions and habits that causes dysbyosis includes chronic stress, low fiber diets, use of antibiotics, chlorinated and fluoridated water, alcoholic beverages, preservatives, soft drinks, and simple carbohydrates like bread, pasta, candy, and fried foods. These substances create conditions that make the bad bugs proliferate and cause all sorts of problems like purification. They eat and break into the walls of the colon and produce systemic circulations, causing chronic degenerative diseases. This is followed by indigestion and the mal-absorption of nutrients required by the immunological building blocks that are supposed to be supplied to the liver. The presence of toxic wastes in the gut causes intestinal toxemia where toxins from the digestive tract poison the blood stream. Dr. Metchnikoff believed that the consumption of cultured fermented diary products that contain probiotic organism was the reason for longevity among Bulgarians.

About 20 years ago, homeostatic soil organisms (HSOs) were discovered in the soil ecosystems where organic plants are grown. They are missing in modern diets due to food processing, pasteurization, isolation, and pesticides. In the soil, HSOs ward off pathogens, maintain homeostatic soil pH, and engulf mold, fungi, and putrefactive bacteria in rotten plant matter. They are able to transform these wastes into nutrients that fertilize and sustain plant life. The inherent abilities they confer to the soil and plant ecosystem are transferred to humans when consumed whole as nature intended. HSOs are our first line of immunological defense. They stimulate T cell activities of the immune system producing proteins the body interprets as antigens. The body sees these proteins as foreign substances and launches an immunological attack against them. These cascading T cells activities ultimately lead to the production of a key immune system regulator, the polypeptide alpha interferon. The T cells similarly stimulate the B lymphocytes to produce unprogrammable or non-specific antigen fighting antibodies. Being non-specific responses, they have not been programmed to overreact, and they modulate the immune responses better. The interferons are part of these non-specific defense systems. This makes the HSOs stimulant huge reservoirs of antibodies which re-educate and refine immune responses to illnesses. Consequently, the immune cells mount necessary but not excessive responses to antigenic response (Rubin, 2002). Probiotic supplements can protect individual with hepatitis B and C from developing liver cancer when they consume food that contain afflatoxins. Foods mostly contaminated with afflatoxins are peanuts, dried figs, spices, and corns. They are produced by molds that grow on food crops during production and storage (Cabot, 1996).

What is glandular reactivation?
The assumption behind management of immune deficiencies with glandular remedies is that "like heals like" such as treating a weak organ with a young fresh healthy portion of the deficient organ. "Within the medical community, any gland that decreases in size or dries up is replaced. If the thyroid dries up, we replace the thyroid. If the pancreas dries up insulin is given to prevent diabetes. If the adrenals dry up, Cortisone is given to prevent Addison's disease. If the ovaries dry up, females are given hormones replacements. If the thymus dries up, it makes equal sense to supplement the thymus or else the immune system suffers. Since cell-mediated immunity and T- cell-mediated immune response are crucial to the eradication of the hepatitis virus, the HIV virus, and cancerous cells, thymus supplementation with thymus gland extract would be a good idea." Carson Burgsteiner MD

Thymus Gland Extracts: Nature's Interferons
If the T cells are the general commanding officer of the immune system, the thymus gland is the "field marshal" of all cell-mediated immunities. Insufficient production of thymic proteins to program the T cells is the etiology of most chronic degenerative diseases and infections. The thymus gland is part of the endocrine and lymphatic systems of the human body, and reaches its maximum size at puberty and gradually begins to shrink as we age. The function of the thymus gland is dependent on its size. Age, disease, stress, toxins, and drugs affect the size and integrity of the thymus gland. The thymus gland plays a prominent role in cell-mediated immunity; it is the booster for all T-cell activities. Without the proteins produced by the thymus gland, the T cells are naïve, immature, and cannot function. The T-helper cells are programmed to identify pathogens in the blood stream, secrete interleukins, and interferons by the actions of proper thymic proteins. Thymus extracts help supplement this deficiency

in function by increasing the numbers and functions of the T cells. It is thought that these cells serve as primary indicators for individuals who are likely to clear the hepatitis virus upon infection. The integrity of the thymus gland helps the T lymphocytes commit themselves, stay vigilant, and protect individuals against specific pathogens for the rest of their as a major constituent of the immune memory.

Thymus extracts are derived from thymus glands of young bovine calves. The *Encyclopedia of Natural Medicine* lists thymus extracts as a treatment for infective hepatitis. It states that there is a good clinical data to support the effectiveness of orally-administered bovine thymus extracts in treating acute and chronic viral hepatitis. It reports the effectiveness of the thymus extract in treating viral hepatitis is reflective of a broad spectrum of immune system enhancements, presumably mediated by improved thymus gland activity (Murray And Pizzorno 1998).

Liver Glandular

Liver extracts from young bovine cows, like its thymic counterpart, help supply the ailing liver with deficient factors necessary for its reactivation; hence they are referred to as glandular reactivation factors. In a diseased state, levels of antioxidants, enzymes, and growth factors are lowered in the liver, the exogenous supply of these factors that are grown in conditions free of hormones, steroids, pesticides, and with unadulterated water can effectively supplement these liver deficiencies. By helping to supply the needed vitamins, enzymes, this young bovine thymic extract from cows grown on free-range farms promotes liver regeneration, and supplies needed protein and enzymes to combat like chronic hepatitis and liver disease.

"Good fortune is what happens when opportunity meets with preparation."

Thomas Edison

Doctors Health Advisory: Because of concerns about mad cow disease, poor sanitary conditions in the slaughter houses, and the liver's function as a store house of toxins, always make sure you are using freeze-dried extracts from young free-range and grass-fed bovine cows.

Chapter 7

Herbal remedies for liver disease

"Modern medicine does not allow for the healing potential inherent in each individual. A program for liver health includes a diet designed to alleviate liver stress or disease, plus an effective herbal formula and other dietary supplements such as antioxidants and essential fatty acids. Such program will cause liver enzymes to return to normal range as well as decreased or low viral load. The liver will get better and a long and a healthy life can be anticipated." Herbalist Christopher Hobbs

How do herbs heal the body?

An orthodox approach to healthcare is a "We care, God heals" approach. The art of healing is a proactive approach instead of the passivity advocated by conventional methods. Hepatitis, as the name implies, is primarily an inflammation and not an infection. The viral loads that conventional medicine uses as its therapeutic yardstick is an effect and not the cause of hepatitis. Just as a plant that flourishes in a favorable soil environment, no matter how much we control its growth, unless we change the soil environment the plant will always flourish. So too with viruses, disease, and cancer cells. When the internal environment is fertile, viruses multiply. As we change our internal environment we reduce our viral loads. The theme of this book is how to change our internal environment. The treatment of infectious hepatitis as an infection to justify expensive orthodox therapy is a medical disgrace. Hepatitis inflammation does not require steroids but dietary factors that reverse cellular inflammation, as explained in Dr. Floyd H. Chilton's book *The War Within*. Viruses are lifeless entities that cannot exist on their own without a favorable internal host environment. The internal environment that favors viral replication is constitutional acidity and fermentation, which in simple English is inflammation. The emphasis on the viral component and the use of antivirals in the management of infective hepatitis is like pouring gasoline on fire. These antiviral drugs increase extracellular matrix toxicity, the launching pad for viral replication. As antiviral remedies engage the viruses, the host body is caught in the ensuring crossfire which manifests as the side effects associated with antiviral use. The adverse reactions associated with drug use are due to their exacerbation of liver inflammation.

In Dr. Strand's book *Death by Prescription*, he points out that "while the Centers For Disease Control estimate that office-based physicians prescribe approximately 100 million courses of antibiotics yearly, viruses do not respond to antibiotics. Ones own immune system will normally get rid of them with time." Ironically, the common cold and stomach viruses that do not respond to any antiviral or antibiotic remedies always depend on the immune system for resolution. Antiviral like Baraclude and Viread that are used to treat infective hepatitis cost above 600 dollars for a 30-day supply. Interferon is in immune system and makes infected cells self destruct. Ironically, synthetic interferon does not have any resemblance to our innate interferons, hence their use is like a delivery van breaking into your front door to deliver you groceries. Since they don't fit the body's chemistry, they cannot launch the immunological response needed for viral clearance. We need to redirect our efforts from attacking the virus to managing the viral environment. Viruses are lifeless creatures that become alive in an inflammatory environment. By addressing inflammation with herbs, detoxification, diets, lifestyle changes, and nutrition, we cut off the supply lines for viral multiplication and consequently reverse liver disease. By clearing the extracellular spaces and lymphatic system of cellular debris and metabolic waste, we strengthen the immune system. By reversing liver inflammation, we optimize immune function which ultimately eradicates the viruses as explained by Doctors Strand and Chilton:

Drug companies are looking for the "silver bullet," or magic cure for liver disease while intentionally neglecting alternative remedies because the gift of nature cannot be patented for corporate profit. Their bottom line is more important than public welfare. Ironically, solutions based on silver-bullets never work as intended in hepatology, agriculture, or any other health science. Penicillin, the gold standard of silver bullets, is now of diminishing usefulness because of widespread development of bacterial strains resistant to it. Like microbes, the hepatitis virus cells develop resistance to newer mono-drug therapies. We need to shift emphasis from the treatment of the disease and attack of the virus to rebuilding the liver, the body, and the immune system. To find lasting solutions to this quagmire, we must shift our mindset to a more holistic approach as has been done in organic farming where primary emphasis is placed on creating an enabling soil environment in which insect pests cannot easily survive in nutrient rich soil. These views are congruent with that of Louis Pastur, the father of the germ theory of disease who on his death bed recounted with these words "I was wrong, the germ is nothing; the terrain is everything." This multifaceted approach builds the health of the soil and attacks the pest from several different angles, which is, the exact opposite of the magic silver-bullet approach of drug-based medicine.

Liver-repair, immune-stimulating, and bile-moving herbs unlock the cell walls via the extracellular matrix, allowing the healing and anti-viral substances to penetrate deep into the nucleus. This creates an opening for botanical anti-viral herbs to move in and mop out the viruses. Detoxification with cleansing herbs guarantee that the dead pathogenic viral agents are eliminated the natural way. Regenerating herbs stimulate and rebuild the extracellular matrix and cells to produce a natural healthy body.

Have you ever wonder why some who are exposed to the infective hepatitis virus do not get infected? The answer lies in the ability of some individuals to effectively clear toxins in the extracellular matrix and pass them on to the lymphatic immune system when antibodies neutralize them. The extracellular matrix (ECM) explains this. This is the space nature put in place between the cells that makes up all of the organs of the human body. It is this space that serves as waiting room for nutrients before they go into the cells where they rebuild our body. It is also a holding room where wastes are retained before being passed to the lymphatic system where they are cleaned and passed back to the general circulation. When wastes are retained for too long in this space, they become a breeding ground for infective and degenerative diseases that plague humanity. Our inability to get rid of cellular waste indicates a weak constitution which in simple language means a weak immune system.

Cellular wastes are different from the solid wastes of the digestive system. For individuals who lack the ability to manage cellular wastes, botanicals and lymph-stimulating nutrients and lifestyles can assist in this process to achieve viral clearance. Different toxins, such as chemicals, heavy metals, viral and bacterial residues, indoor pollutants (e.g. gases from carpet and paints), diet, antibiotics, and other drugs residues are stored in the ECM, because they are so harmful to the cells. Given enough time the toxins *exceed* the storage capacity of ECM and impair the ability for the body to regulate and regenerate. Rapidly, non-specific symptoms emerge, e.g. fatigue, headache, muscular pain, mood swings, and allergies. Your immune-lymphatic system shuts down. It can no longer compensate for the toxic overload within you and leaves you a sitting duck for all kinds of viruses, bacteria, and other microbes to move in. This viscous cycle continues as your now-toxic body is actually turned into a playground for these unwanted guests. They are having the time of their life at your expense.

First, we need to get you back to natural health by "cleansing" yourself from the inside, allowing your body to reset, and heal itself by stopping once and for all the incessant attacks on your extracellular matrix.

Through the actions of herbs in the liver, we can turn the tables in our favor and make viruses play by our rules. The liver-shield herbs change our internal environment to one of natural health, literally unlocking our health from the inside out. What's more, not only do these herbs make us feel amazing, they create an environment so repulsive and uninhabitable for the viruses within us that they wave the white flag. This uninhabitable environment forces the viruses to retreat. We have now essentially changed the rules.

⊠ *Flashback*
Detoxifications with herbal retentions and coffee enemas, nutrition with fortified green drinks, bile-moving herbs, lymphatic herbs, herbal blood cleansers including milk thistle , herbal antibiotics described in Stephen Buhner's book, far-infrared saunas, lymphatic drainage, and lifestyle modifications made my prognosis favorable, along with positive seroconversion. By reducing the toxic load off my liver, it repaired itself and overwhelmed the hepatitis virus.

In contrast to conventional antivirals, we propose a four-pronged, multi-faceted, result-based approach with herbal and naturopathic remedies using the following protocol: *"Even if you are on the right track, you'll get run over if you just sit there."*
Will Rogers

- Relieve the liver's toxic load with detoxifications and bile moving herbs.
- Strengthen the cellular integrity and immune systems with botanical supplements to prevent viral entrance and penetration, i.e. repair and regeneration of damaged liver cells.
- Control viral replication with botanical antibiotics.
- Control dietary imbalances that fuel the excessive inflammatory messengers to ensure that appropriate immunological signals are sent.

What herbs should I stay away from without qualified supervision?
The simple answer is all herbs that are not recommended by a qualified herbalist, naturopath, or other qualified alternative and orthodox healthcare practitioner. The following is a partial list:

- Ephedra and Chinese Ephedra,
- Atractylis Gummifera,
- Ma Huang,
- Azadirachza indica,
- Beriberis vulgaris,
- Callilepsis laureola,
- Cassia angustifolia (senna),
- Crotalaria, Corydalis,
- Hedeoma pulegoides,
- Heliotropium,
- Larrea tridenata (Chaparral bush, Creosote bush, Grease wood),
- Lycopodium serratum (Jin Bu Huan),
- Mentha pulegoides,
- Sassafras albidum (Sassafras),
- Scuteileria (Skull cap),
- Stephania,
- Symphytum officinale (Comfrey),
- Teucrium chamaedrys,
- Tussilago farfara (peppermint),
- Valeriana oficinalis (Valerian, Asfetida, Hops, Genitian),
- Viscum alba (Mistletoe),
- Margosa oil,

- Mate tea,
- Godololobo yerba tea,
- Pennyroyal (squawmint oil),
- Senecio,
- Heliotropium,
- Chelidonum majus (greater celandine),
- Artemisia,
- Hare's ear,
- Chrysanthemum,
- Plantago seed,
- Gardina,
- Red Peony root

What should I avoid for my liver to heal?
- Alcohol,
- Medications with alcohol
- Shellfish (oysters and clams; they increase the risk of bepatitis A and bacteria vibrio vulnificus)
- Wild mushrooms; they might contain the toxins phalloidin and alpha amanintin
- Saccharin
- Aflatoxin
- Tap water
- Cow milk and diary products,
- Isolated Vitamins A, D and niacin,
- High iron multivitamin supplements,
- Carbonated drinks,
- Over-the-counter medications,
- Anger, envy, jealousy and chronic stress,
- Cleaning solutions containing alcohol, isopropyl alcohol and sodium hydrochloride,
- Synthetic yard supplies, e.g. fertilizers, yard sprays, bug sprays etc,
- Household paints,
- Smoke and exhaust,
- General environmental pollutants from paint thinners and aerosol sprays,
- Caffeine; replace caffeine with herbal teas

When inhaled, environmental pollutants are passed to the liver via the lungs and discharged into the bile. It is important to control exposure to control liver damage. Similarly, it is advisable to use gloves, cover the skin, or wash off any chemicals that you come in contact with. Clean blood spills with bleach.

☒ *Flashback*
I allowed a time lapse of several hours between conventional drugs and herbal remedies, and I tried as much as possible to start herbal remedies at lower doses, working my way up, while watching for hypersensitivity and allergic reactions. I followed the principle developed by the father of homeopathic Medicine, Dr Samuel Hahnemann, who in 1796 proposed that "infinitesimal doses of remedies will produce better healing results than the larger doses."

For healing to take place, bio-synergertic compatibility is required. The life span of the liver cells is about 18 months. We anticipate an average of six months of disciplined effort on the part of liver patients to begin to see results. Only plant remedies that are bio-synergistically compatible with the human body can elicit healing. Since drugs are not compatible with human biochemistry, they never elicit healing. Our biochemical make up constantly generates information that points to what is going on in our body if we just listen to our body. Alternative remedies are a journey. Our individual requirements for excellent health are both physically and mentally different. Our physical and mental tolerances are different. Our dosage requirements are also different. Our allergic responses to different herbs vary, too.

"By combining the best that traditional medicine has to offer and incorporating healthy lifestyles, everyone has the best chance of protecting his health."-Ray Strand MD

Safety issues associated with botanicals

Herbal remedies should be approached with the same caution as with conventional drugs, especially in individuals taking synthetic drugs because of herb – drug interactions. Individuals taking diuretics need to be particularly careful with herbs with high potassium content. One of the main problems with assessing natural products for health benefits is the lack of good clinical trial data. Most of the evidence is, at best, anecdotal involving the uncontrolled use of products of unknown quality. There is no doubt that many of these traditional "medicines" are biologically active and, by a process of natural selection, may be beneficial. However, like pharmaceutical products, the beneficial effects are likely to be dose-dependent, and it is likely that these active agents will have a spectrum of biological activity that may cause toxicity. Without good clinical trial data and with no quality control of the product, it is unlikely these agents will consistently provide therapeutic benefit.

Beware of herb-drug interactions

According to Michael Tierra, author of the book The Way of Herbs, *"herbal remedies take the body through three phases: eliminating and detoxifying, maintaining health by healing the body of physical symptoms and finally building the body by toning the organs. If one is undergoing herbal therapy for an extended period of time, it must be understood that the body, as with everything else in nature, functions cyclically with a period of maximum effectiveness in the use of herbs and that effectiveness is benefited by regular breaks. Dr Tierra recommends one day break for every seven days of use of herbs. This gives the body the needed rest and preparing it to respond with renewed vigor.*

Alternative remedies, like drugs, are not "one size fits all." To discover what is best for us, we need to start with lower doses and work up. While we get immediate responses from synthetic drugs, herbs work only after they have established themselves in the body and developed synergy with our biochemistry. Only buy herbs from trusted, reputable, reliable sources, and always check botanical plant names to be sure you are buying the correct plant material. Many different plants share the same common names. Start simple, one herb at a time, before trying herbal combinations. This makes it much easier to eliminate herbs to which you might be allergic or sensitive, or those you might simply dislike. It will be very difficult to pinpoint an herbal allergy from a preparation containing five different herbs. Organic is best. If you are using fresh herbs in your preparations, double the quantity of the amount stated for dried herb(s). Water used in herbal preparations should be free from fluoride and chlorine. Make sure you have a small accurate scale on hand when making herbal preparations. Our bodies constantly generate information that points to what is going on in our body if we listen to our body. Our dosage requirements are also different, and our allergic responses to different herbs vary.

Herbal remedies are definitely not as dramatic as drugs when used under professional supervision. They elicit fewer side effects. But because, like drugs, they block some enzymatic reactions to elicit therapeutic their effects, they can have adverse reactions like pharmaceutical agents (Strand, 2003). Like drugs, when we take any combinations of drugs that utilize the same enzyme systems, bottle necks and back ups are created. This is what is responsible for some of the hypersensitivity of allergic reactions associated with herbs. This is also expected when drugs and herbs utilize the same enzyme systems.

Be aware of your biochemical individuality
Each individual has a unique constitution that favors the right mix of nutrients. We differ in the quantities of nutrients we each need to attain health. One man's remedy can be another man's poison. An excellent remedy for your auntie might be your nightmare. We differ in food preferences which reflect our biochemical and physiological differences. We need to pay attention to how different remedies, herbs and nutrient impart and affect our energy levels, moods, and body (Brinker, 2001). It takes a determined effort and a willing heart to change established mental and physical factors that made us ill. If we are not cognizant of the physiological signals generated within our body regarding illness, we begin a process that removes our awareness from our own nature. We end up making poor lifestyle choices that gradually results in physical degeneration. What is good for us depends more on what our body needs than expert opinion. It took a long time for our bodies to become receptive to diseases to set in, and it will take equal diligence and patience for us to make our internal environments defy illness (Erasmus, 1993).

While the FDA tests and regulate the quality, sale, and distribution of drugs, manufacturers of alternative remedies are not required by law to prove to the FDA that that their products are effective and safe for human consumption as long as they do not claim that they can prevent, cure, and treat any illness. Some alternative remedies have been found to not contain the amount of remedies stated on their labels and some may contain impurities and contaminants. Also, the actual amounts advertised may differ among brands or different batches of the same brand. Most of the available alternative remedies have not been evaluated for their interactions with drugs, foods and other remedies, either.

Most of the alternative remedies available were not produced in the United States and are presumed not to meet FDA standards. Consequently, people whose cancer are declared terminal and want alternative remedies that are suppressed by the FDA go by the thousands to Europe and South America and are coming back home healed. While alternative medicine is based of promise and word of mouth, orthodox approaches have historical analysis, double-blind studies, and placebo-controlled studies to back their approaches. Alternative remedies are not scientifically evaluated, making it hard to identify charlatans taking advantage of vulnerable patients.

Please avoid herbs that are imported from other countries because of the following reasons.
- The conditions under which the herbs are grown may be questionable.
- Their regulatory agencies, like the FDA, are heavily manipulated by herb manufacturers.
- Labeling errors frequently occur with herbal medicines, and often times, substitutions are made in traditional imported herbal remedies. It is important to use only imported herbs that are recommended for a specific condition by an herbalist or a reputable practitioner who is experienced with herbs and your condition.

If you experience a negative change in your body or you experience a new set of symptoms when taking any herb or medication, always think of a potential adverse drug reaction first (Strand, 2003). Common adverse reactions that should warrant discontinuation of herbal remedies includes skin rashes, nausea, bloating, fatigue, aching in the liver area, yellowing of the skin, and/or pale feces (Cohen, Gish and Doner, 2001).

Websites to check for possible drug-herb and drug-drug interactions
http://www.aafp.org/afp/20080101/73.html
http://www.itmonline.org/arts/herbdrug2.htm
http://www.i-care.net/herbdrug.htm
http://www.healthcastle.com/herb_drugfood.shtml
http://www.nlm.nih.gov/medlineplus/druginfo/natural/patient

http://www.drugdigest.org/wps/portal/ddigest

"Men are not disturbed by things that happen but by their opinion of the things that happen." Eepictetus

Which herbal doses do I start with?

The key to good herbal remedies is to use fresh, high-quality, organic herbs. When purchasing the herbs, do not simply choose any brand off the store shelf. Be sure it contains organic, recently-harvested quality herbs. You may be surprised at the quality of herbs being sold to unsuspecting consumers. Consultation with an herbalist who knows how to determine quality is highly recommended. It is best to find the bulk herbs that have not been processed.

Properties of individual medicinal herbs
http://www.naturalark.com/
http://www.altnature.com/gallery/
http://www.nlm.nih.gov/medlineplus/druginformation.html
http://www.naturalstandard.com/
http://www.herballegacy.com/index.html
http://www.medicinehunter.com/
http://plants.usda.gov/java/profile?symbol=asal7

How to become your own Herbalist

Always use stainless steel pots, Pyrex bowls, earthenware, or enamel cookware, free from chips and cracks. Aluminum cookware can react with the chemicals in the herb and affect the end product. Aluminum is also known to accumulate in the body over time and has been implicated in Alzheimer's disease. Hygiene is important when preparing herbs for medicines, particularly if you intend to store the preparations. Sterilize all jars and bottles. This can be done by boiling them and their lids separately for 20 minutes or putting them in an oven and heating them to 350°F for one hour. They can also be sterilized if soaked in bleach for about one hour and then rinsed of with clean water.

The website www.livershield.net offers a wide range of botanical remedies and supplements for liver diseases, fatty liver, hepatitis C, hepatitis B, liver gallbladder flush and detoxifications.

How to Capsulate Herbs and Herb Formulas

Mix the herbal combinations in the dosage and quantity desired, and grind them into powdered from with a coffee grinder. (For electric coffee grinders, we recommend the Cuisinart coffee bean grinder.) Powdered herbs can be used directly with fruit or vegetable juices, in shakes, or put into capsules. Money can be saved and quality guaranteed when you buy herbs in bulk (by the pound) or in powdered form, and put them into capsules yourself using a homemade encapsulator or a by-hand capsule machine that can be bought from a local health food store or over the Internet.

Capsulation is also helpful because enzymes may be lost when we make herbal teas. Also, it is often difficult to swallow bitter herbs in raw form. The blank "0" capsule and a capsule machine that houses the single "0" capsule size can be used. When capsulating a formula of herbs, combine the herbs in the proper amounts, mix thoroughly, and capsulate. It is that simple. If you chose to use the larger "00" capsule size, make sure you buy the "00" capsule machine. The capsule machine is cheaper than what you will spend on a lunch date.

If you choose to make your own capsules, we suggest you use a by-hand capsule machine like the "Cap-M-Quick" from www.cap-m-quick.com. You can also get your gelatin capsules from this company.

Alkaloid and medicinal properties of herbal teas
When we say herbal teas, we don't imply basic tea but infusions and/or decoctions.

Tea is an important dietary source of flavanols. Tea polyphenols may possess the bioactivity to affect the pathogenesis of several chronic diseases, especially cardiovascular disease and cancer. Herbal teas can selectively destroy diseased cells while nourishing healthy cells. These alkaloids or secondary compounds in tea, called catechins, have potent anti-oxidant properties which help reduce the risk of disease by fixing cell damage.

Among other roles, catechins have been shown to inhibit growth of diseased cells and to keep them from spreading to other parts of the body. Tea is the best source of catechins in the human diet. Teas are quickly absorbed into the body where they exert their therapeutic effects, especially in people with liver disease.

Supplement makers have responded to the positive results of tea research with a multitude of tea extracts. Perhaps the most popular, epigallocatechin gallate (EGCG), is popping up in a variety of nutritional supplements, from multivitamins to herbal concoctions. Though EGCG may have some benefit, it should be used in moderation. Very high amounts of green tea components have been shown to interact with drugs that affect blood clotting, such as aspirin, and also may cause liver damage.

Make Tea a Part of Your Diet
Some studies found that people who drink 6 cups of tea daily realized maximum health benefits. However, some studies show health benefits, including liver disease prevention, in only 1 to 4 cups of tea daily. Choosing the correct form of tonic is also important. Brewed tea, either hot or iced, offers the most potent disease-fighting activity. Instant iced tea and bottled tea beverages offer little health benefit.

The key to realizing the potential health benefits of tea is consistency. Consumed regularly over many years, white, green, and black teas can offer substantial protection against liver diseases and infective hepatitis. When combined with a mostly plant-based diet, the catechins from tea could have an even greater effect, as all the plant chemicals work together to safeguard health. This is the power of synergy.

Basic Tea Recipe
- 1 ounce dried herbs
- ½ pint water

Place herbs into a clean non-reactive metal or enamel pot with a lid. Bring water to a boil. Turn off the heat and pour the water over the herb(s). Cover the pot and let steep for 5 – 10 minutes. Strain using a non-aluminum strainer and drink. Honey, lemon, or milk can be added if desired.

Herbal Infusions

An infusion is often stronger than a tea and will extract glycosides, alkaloid salts, water-soluble vitamins, and volatile oils. Infusions are intended for immediate use. They can be stored for a maximum of 24 hours in a cool place.

Basic Infusion Recipe
- 1 ounce of dried herbs
- 1 pint boiling water

Pour water of herbs. Steep for 10 – 20 minutes then strain and drink. Sweeten if desired.

DECOCTIONS

This method is used for hard woody substances such as roots, bark, and stems whose constituents are water soluble and non-volatile. A decoction is used to extract minerals, bitter components, etc. from hard materials such as roots, bark or seeds by boiling for a few minutes and then allowing the herbs to steep for several hours Decoctions are also intended for immediate use. Store for a maximum of 72 hours in a very cool place.

Basic Decoction Recipe
- 1 oz of dried herb or root
- 1 pint water

Cut or crush herb or root and add to water. Simmer with the lid off until the volume of water is reduced by ¼, so ¾ of a pint remains. Cool, strain, and separate in divided doses according to the herb's use. Sweeten if desired.

TINCTURES

Tinctures extract the chemical constituents in alcohol cider vinegar or vegetable glycerin. (White vinegar is synthetic and defeats the purpose.),

Alcohol is most effective and therefore the most commonly used. *In children and individuals with liver disease or alcoholics, alcohol-based extracts are contraindicated*. Vinegar or vegetable glycerin can be used where there is a reason not to use alcohol. Tinctures are invaluable, as water will retrieve only some of the medicinal properties. You can certainly use 90 percent or higher alcohol for any tincture, but to save money, find out required alcohol concentration for each herb. For example, garlic requires only 25 percent alcohol, while Chaste Tree berries require 75 percent.

Tinctures are extremely useful, quick, easy, simple to dispense, and will last indefinitely if stored correctly. They are also a good substitute if an infusion or decoction is too bitter to drink.

Basic Tincture Recipe
- 1 – 2 ounces of powdered or chopped herb
- 1 pint of alcohol such as vodka, cider vinegar, or vegetable glycerin

Mix herb with liquid. Keep the tincture in a tightly closed jar in a warm spot (but not in the sun), for approximately 2 weeks. Shake the tincture 2 to 3 times every day. Strain through a coffee filter, folded cheesecloth, or muslin. You may need to strain your tincture two or even three times to remove the entire herb.

Store your tincture in a dark bottle or cabinet. Half a pint of tincture should equal the medicinal potency of 1 ounce of the fresh herb, so approx. 1 t. will equal the medicinal strength of 1 cup of infusion. Dilute at least 1 t. of tincture in ¼ cup of water.

To make ground herbs, pour all herbs into a bowl, shake thoroughly, and grind with coffee grinder. Add 4 parts of ground organic flax seed. Mix with super green foods and take two table spoons twice daily in juice, shake or water

What is an herbal tonic?
An herbal tonic is a preparation of one or multiple herbs. In this chapter, we will be dealing with ground herbs, capsulation, tinctures, decoctions, and infusions. A good resource to check for the medicinal properties of medicinal herbs is to use the search words "herbal database" in any of the search engines in the Internet.

Make ground herbs, infusions, or decoctions of the following liver-shield herbs, and make sure that most of these herbs are not on the FDA hit lists. Have you wondered why you are told to stay away from botanical herbs and supplements but to take botanical fruits and vegetables? With moderation, the use of these herbs can help you live your life without liver disease. When the government determines that your condition is terminal, they have inadvertently lost jurisdiction over your desire to use alternative remedies to regain your health.

Blood tonics clean the blood of toxins and metabolic wastes that feed viral multiplication or perpetuate cirrhotic damage. By eliminating wastes, there are more oxygen carrying capacities for the hemoglobin. Viruses cannot replicate in oxygen-rich blood. As we cleanse the blood, we increase its alkalinity and change cellular metabolism from fermentation to oxidation. We ultimately reduce the viral load

Herbal tonics for liver disease, hepatitis C and hepatitis B

- Delight yourself with this nutritious blood tonic with the following formulation: 1 part of red clover, 5 parts of Burdock root, 1 part of Poke root, 2 parts of Yellow dock root, 1½ parts of Goldenseal root, 2 parts of Oregon grape root, 1 part of Bloodroot, and 4 parts of Licorice root.
- Make an effective lymphatic-immune tonic with the following formulation: 1 part of Red root, 4 parts of Burdock, 5 parts of Cleavers, 2 parts of Yellow Duck, 5 parts of Calendula, ½ part of Stinging nettles, ½ part Sassafras, and 1 part of Red clover,
- Make a nourishing liver repair and bile tonic with the following formulation: 4 parts of Astragulus,5 parts of Licorice, 5 parts of Burdock, 3 parts of Artichoke, 3 parts Echinacea purpora, 4 parts of Dandelion, 3 parts of Oregon grape root, and 4 parts of Turmeric

Stephen Harrods's book *Herbal Antibiotics* lists a wide variety of botanicals that create internal environments that are unfavorable to microbial proliferation. Make anti-microbial capsules with the following: 4 parts Garlic, 4 parts Echinacea purpora, 5 parts Aloe vera, 3 parts Golden seal, 3 parts Grapefruit seed extract, 3 parts Ginger, 2 parts Sage, including 5 parts Olive leaf (because it is bitter), and 5 parts Milk thistle (because it is not water soluble)

- If it is cumbersome to do these herbs individually, this combination encompasses the whole herb. Make decoctions, infusions, capsulations, and ground herbal tonics with the following: 3 parts of Artichoke, 2 parts of Astragulus, 4 Parts of Burdock, 4 parts of Calendula, 5 parts of Milk thistle, 5 parts of Turmeric, 5 parts of Olive leaf, 3parts of ground flax seed, 2 parts of Yellow Duck, 3 parts of Oregon grape Root, 3 parts of Cleavers, 5 parts of Burdock root, 1 part of Goldenseal root, 3 parts of Licorice root, and 3 parts Ginger root.

Miscellaneous Notes

- Discard used herbs. Refrigerate tea. Suggested use: Take ½ to 1 cup of prepared formula tea 2 – 3 times a day; take a 2-week break and repeat. Take another 2-week break and repeat again.
- Alternate the infusions and/or decoctions with two tablespoons of ground herb mixed with 3 parts of ground organic flax seeds. Take 2 teaspoons twice daily in water, organic fruit or vegetable juices, green drinks, or shakes.
- The body must be able to eliminate unhealthy cells and dead matter from the body. You should have a bowel movement at least 2 – 3 times a day. If you are not, increase the amount of times you take the formula. However, you also do not want to induce diarrhea. If you do, decrease the amount of each dose and/or how often you take it.
- Using any of the above formulas may make you weak if your body is already fragile and/or you have had orthodox treatments. These recipes have powerful herbs that draw chemicals and poisons from your tissues in order to eliminate them. Sometimes it is too much for a frail body to take all at once. Use it wisely. Ease off, and then try again.
- Finally, it may not be advisable to use the lymphatic and blood cleansers separately. A whole-body cleanse that includes individual discretion in selecting 2 – 3 herbs from each group to make a whole-body herbal cleanse may be advisable. However, if a decision is made to use the herbs separately wait a week before switching to cleansing another organ.

How Dr. Peter Oyakhire used the herbal protocol with lifestyle changes to manage cancer, hepatitis B, and liver cirrhosis

Studies show that for every year of having masquerading symptoms before a chronic degenerative disease diagnosis, we need an average of one month of aggressive alternative treatment. Generally, these remedies will start a detoxification process of getting rid of established old patterns, opening the eliminative channels before healing can begin to take place

Though my de-compensated cirrhosis is thought to be non-reversible, the progression to cancer can be stopped if individuals modify their lifestyles. I knew that for me to keep liver cancer at bay, heal my cancer, stop cirrhotic degeneration of my liver, and keep my viral load from hepatitis B to undetectable , I had to do bi-weekly coffee or herbal-retention enemas or quarterly colonics to take the load off of my liver, eliminate red meat from my diet, consume free-range organic chicken and wild-caught sea food, replace table salt with rock salt or sea salt, replace white sugar with raw honey or raw brown sugar sparingly, replace white bread with whole wheat bread or sourdough bread, stop taking alcoholic beverages, do not use tobacco, stay away from non-prescription drugs, stay away from tap water, replace cow's milk with goat milk, rice milk and soy milk, stay away from carbonated drinks, take milk thistle and olive leaf extract daily, drink 6 – 8 glasses of purified water and/or juices daily, maintain excellent digestive health, replace hydrogenated oils, vegetable oils, and trans fatty acids with organic cold-pressed extra virgin olive oil and coconut oil, stay away from fast foods and fried foods, exercise regularly to reduce glucose (sugar) demands of cancer cells, and cheat occasionally on all of the above. I regularly consumed decoctions made primarily from the cancer and liver tonic herbs. I consumed food combinations that have a 1-to-2 protein-to-carbohydrate ratio, and a 70: 30 raw- to-cooked food ratio.

The fortified green drinks are commercially-prepared powerful blends of enzyme-rich nutrients and antioxidant-rich super foods which supply an impressive ORC (oxygen-radical absorbance capacity) assay which measures anti-oxidant capacity against cell damaging free radicals that would otherwise break down healthy cells and lead to a variety of degenerate diseases. These drinks supply organically-grown, wild–crafted, nutrient-rich greens that naturally supply vitamins, minerals, and amino acids. They must also contain fruit blends that supply phytonutrients, which are the brightly-colored pigments that protect plants from the potentially damaging effects of sunlight and environmental hazards. With my coffee grinder, I ground my herbs with flax seeds, mix them in organic orange juice, and fortified powdered green food. I take two table spoons twice daily. By mixing liver, botanical antibiotics, and cancer tonic as a base for fortified green drinks, I get the best of herbalism and nutrition. This is the basis of daily detoxification for cellular regeneration. I had more good days that bad days, less metabolic crises, and my multitude of symptoms were reduced to zero. My fast-growing aggressive lymphoma was slowed down to a crawl and tumor size was reduced to bean shape sizes. My viral load became undetectable. My hydrocel shrinks and my hernia pains are drastically reduced. I made a metabolic shift from disease crises to de-tox crises. Cancer doesn't scare me any more, but healing crises do as I lost my illness and gained my health.

Milk Thistle: The Liver Mechanic

Milk thistle as a liver remedy is the "gold standard" in the management of all degenerative liver diseases when it comes to rebuilding the terrains of the liver. Milk thistle, also known as silybum marianum, is a member of the daisy family and is related to other thistles. Silybum is the only member of the thistles that contain silymarin, the active ingredient in milk thistle. Silymarin is the collective name by which the primary groups of active isomers of silybin are known. The isomers are silybin, silydianin, and silychristin.

⊠ *Flashback*
The viruses were clearly ravaging my liver and my whole body without any resistance or hindrance on my part. Chemotherapy took away my resistance. Six months into my infection, the doctors determined that I was a chronically-infected patient. The implication of this is that I would have to live with the virus for the rest of my life, and since the medications I was prescribed were not working, I was told to go home and die or live with hepatitis B for the rest of my life. Milk thistle was my fortress! It saved my life. It helped repair instead of replace my liver through transplantation. It took me permanently away from the surgeon's knife. It helped normalized all my liver enzymes to within normal ranges within five months, reversed cirrhotic progression, increased my liver capacity from less than 10 percent to more than 60 percent, regenerated damaged tissue, cleared my jaundice, ascites, hepatic encephalopathy, and increased my vigor. Hurray!!! Milk thistle did not do it alone; I worked effectively with my lifestyle changes.

Silymarin is subjected to enterohepatic circulation, an intestinal-to-liver loop. It moves from the blood to the bile and is concentrated in the liver cells. This cycle is difficult to break and it makes the herb very effective. Like the windjammer, milk thistle gives the liver stability and strength by stopping the entrance of toxins. It inhibits the factors that are responsible for hepatic damage like free radicals. Milk thistle does prevent death to the liver cells at a cost much far lower than standard drug remedies. It facilitates formation of new liver proteins that are incorporated into the cell walls of the liver hepatocytes. This makes them stronger and resistant to the entrance of toxins. By increasing the rate of protein synthesis, it facilitates liver regeneration. Silymarin inhibits the production of the enzymes that produce substances that can damage the liver. It prevents the depletion of glutathione on the liver, hepatocytes. Glutathione mediates liver-cell metabolism. These have anti-oxidant properties. The mechanism for Silymarin's protein synthesis in liver cells is a result of increased activity of ribosomal RNA via the nuclear polymerase A. The ribosomes are cellular organelles where protein synthesis takes place. The silybin molecule has a part-steroid structure. Steroids enter the cell and stimulate the induction of new DNA and ribosomal RNA synthesis (Hobbs, 2002).

These facts are corroborated by Dr. Andrew Well, director of the integrative medicine program at the university of Arizona, with the following quote: *"The pharmaceutical industry offers nothing to match the protective effect of milk thistle which itself is non-toxic…I recommend this herb to all patients with chronic hepatitis, abnormal liver function, and have seen cases of normalization of liver functions in persons who took it everyday for several months and worked to improve their diets and lifestyles…If you are already a heavy user of alcohol, pharmaceutical drugs (including cancer patients on chemotherapy), or have been exposed to toxic chemicals from any source, take milk thistle…It will help your body recover from any harm."*

Control of Hepatitis Viruses with Herbal Antibiotics
"The relationship between viral load and liver [cell] damage is the subject of great professional controversy. Alternative modalities emphasize evaluations that monitor the response of the host body to the hepatitis C virus over how much virus is in the liver. This approach stresses that the body's constitutional make-up determines the immune response to the infection and has more influence than the viral load in determining how much inflammatory damage has been done. Lifestyles, dietary, and environmental factors play greater roles in promoting the progression of liver disease than the viral count." Howard Monsour, M.D.

Olive leaf Extract: Nature's Antibiotic

The pharmaceutical industry has not been able to come up with a non-toxic antiviral that can engage the hepatitis virus without endangering the individual. Olive leaf extract can! It is the most versatile non-prescription anti-microbial remedy nature has provided for humanity. Unlike antibiotic plants that predate human existence, the pharmaceutical industries produce newer anti-virals every six months because the viruses keep altering their shapes to elude the anti-virals. Lactic acidosis is a life-threatening complication of reverse transcriptase anti-viral drugs used in the management of hepatitis B and C viral infections. Olive leaf extract can eradicate the hepatitis B, C, and HIV viruses with non-toxic consequences and added side benefits. In its natural habitat, the olive leaf controls pest infestations to the extent that commensal relations are maintained; the ecosystem remains intact and its survival is ensured. These capabilities of the olive leaf are retained when humans consume them. While they reduce the viral load to human tolerance, they do not hamper the activities of beneficial microbes in the human body.

Dr. H.E. Remis, a virologist working for the Upjohn Pharmaceutical Company, tried to isolate oleuropein, one of the active ingredients in the olive leaf without success. While oleuropin was found to be virucidal against all viruses *in vitro*—in the test tube—the success did not extend to *in vivo*—in animal studies. *In vivo*, calcium elongate, the active ingredient in olive leaf, quickly bound to proteins in the blood and which rendered it ineffective against viruses. Upjohn came to a business decision to abandon the olive leaf project because they were unable to isolate the active ingredient *in vivo*.

In simple English, the pharmaceutical industry refused to continue the olive leaf project because they could not patent a synthetic version of the natural product.

How do herbs kill microbes (viruses, bacteria, fungi and parasites)?

The conventional management of infective hepatitis is analogous to other infective diseases. Adefovior, a nucleotide ester prodrug was originally evaluated for the treatment of HIV disease. While it is currently referred to by its trade name Preveon, the FDA has informed the manufacturer (Gilead) that a different trade name should be adopted due to conflict with a different product before it can be used for the treatment of infective hepatitis. In his book 'Death By Diet', Robert Barefoot points out that the common HIV drug AZT was initially used as a chemotherapy drug for cancer in the 1960's.He see no justification why drugs meant for a particular diseases can have off label uses for other illness which are sometimes unrelated. The question that begs for answer is, do we really need antimicrobial drugs to manage infective diseases?

In their book, 'Ten Lies About AIDS', Etienne De Harven and Jean-Claude Roussez point out that HIV infection is not the cause of AIDS. Severe immune deficiencies, commonly referred to as AIDS, result from the toxicity of many recreational drugs and of most antiretroviral medications, from the abuse of antibiotics and certain therapeutic protocols, from inappropriate life style, and/or from malnutrition, alone or combined.

In her book, 'Goodbye AIDS! Did it ever exist', Maria Papagiannidou-St Pierre, a senior Greek journalist and ex-AIDS patient thought otherwise. Born in 1965, she was diagnosed "HIV positive" in 1985. From 1995 to 2005 she was a full-blown AIDS patient suffering horrifically from the side-effects of the medications, being sometimes told she had no more than a week to live. In 2006 she started the website www.hivwave.gr and married the Canadian "HIV negative" Gilles St Pierre. In 23 April 2007 she stopped taking the pills prescribed against AIDS, became strong again and regained the freedom we all lost in 1984. So, what had she suffered from, a deadly hoax? She began to research what had happened to her, met many who had questioned the HIV/AIDS dogma on her way, found the missing answers and now wants to shout out around the world: "The elaborate AIDS construction is built on a false foundation!"

In Dr. Simeon Hein's review of the book 'Why We Will Never Win The War On AIDS', He points out how Ellison and Duesberg present a compelling argument that modern medical health organizations have their own interests at heart when it comes to diagnosing and treating infectious diseases. At the end the of the 1960's most infectious diseases like Polio had been eradicated in the western world. This threatened the budgets of federal health agencies the like the CDC and NIH who thrive on public funding to combat transmittable diseases. Cancer seemed like a promising candidate for their research but turned out not to be caused by viruses or microbes.

Dr Hein indicates that when a new disease called AIDS appeared, it provided the promise of huge amounts of funding if it proved to be transmittable. Ellison and Duesberg argue that the health establishment manipulated public perception about the relationship between AIDS and HIV, to create the appearance of a direct linkage, so as to create a new research and health-care paradigm: one that put them at the center of the action. In reality, the vast majority of retroviruses are harmless and AIDS shows very different symptoms depending on which country it appears in. African AIDS is a different beast altogether from that which appears in Europe and the U.S.A... This suggests AIDS isn't one disease but many immune system disorders that have been lumped together under one rubric for the sake of the organizations that specialize in their treatment. According to the authors, anytime someone tests positive for HIV and have any of over 100 symptoms, they are automatically classified as having "AIDS." And yet apparently, many people who test positive for HIV stay healthy for decades.

He shows how Ellison and Duesberg present a lifestyle explanation for what causes AIDS including drug-use, immune system stress, and sexual preference. This is a more sociological driven idea of what AIDS is than a biological explanation. And it challenges everything we've officially been told about the disease.

He summarizes by saying that 'the information presented was an important event in my personal understanding of how scientific institutions actually work, what drives their research, and causes them to sometimes act like witch-hunting "knowledge monopolies." If you are at all interested in the collusion between science, government health policy, and the medical establishment you are bound to find it provocative and challenging.'

Is Hepatitis, like AIDS a "fake epidemic"? Is the immune system stupid? Let's find out.

Historically, plants have provided a good source of anti-infective agents like emetine, quinine, and berberine remain highly effective instruments in the fight against microbial infections. Phytomedicines derived from plants have shown great promise in the treatment of intractable infectious diseases including opportunistic HIV, hepatitis viruses and wide varieties of Sexually transmitted diseases.

During microbial attack or at injury sites, plants secrete resinous substances like lignin, callose, gums, suberin etc which close the site of injury. This is similar to how blood clot prevents bleeding and tissues damage in humans.

Antimicrobial agents like lysozyme and other lytic enzymes in plants can degrade cell wall of microbes and kill them. Plants also produce protease inhibitors which inhibit microbial proteases that serve as life wire for the survival of microbes like the hepatitis viruses, HIV viruses, bacteria, fungi and parasites. Plants also produce secondary metabolites with antimicrobial properties. These secondary compounds include many phenolics (e.g. flavonoids, isoflavones and simple phenolics), glucosinolates, cyanogenic glycosides, acids, aldehydes, saponins, triterpenes and other alkaloids

In his book Alkaloids Secrets of Life, Tadeusz Aniszewski point out that alkaloids, represent a group of interesting and complex chemical compounds, produced by the secondary metabolism of living organisms in different biotopes. They are relatively common chemicals in all kingdoms of living organisms in all environments.

Higher plants produce divergent compounds like alkaloids, terpenoids and phenolic compounds in secondary metabolism. Among these compounds, alkaloids are very important due to their high biological activity. Alkaloids are low molecular weight nitrogen containing compounds that are found in about 25% of plant species and almost all herbs. This lay credence to the fact that herbs have more potent disease fighting capabilities that vegetable and fruit juices. Most alkaloids are produced from amines produced by the decarboxylation of amino acids such as histidine, lysine, ornithine, tryptophan and tyrosine. Because these amino acids as plant derived proteins are the building block of plant alkaloids.

Alkaloids as plant proteins are used to rebuild diseased organs when we are facing chronic organ degenerations like cancer, liver disease, pancreas in diabetes and other tissue assaults during disease. They are synergistically comparable to human tissues compared to animal proteins when regeneration and recovery is required.

Microbes like plants have intelligence to continue to survive. Because synthetic ant-microbial remedies do not have life in them, microbes are able to sense their presence and alter their shape and nomenclature to evade their attack. This ultimately leads to mutants and drug resistant species. This does not happen with botanicals because they have innate intelligence that work bio synergistically with human body to the detriment of microbes. The incompatibility of drugs with microbes and human biochemistry is the cause of the adverse reaction associated with their use.

Botanicals like the olive leaf, Oregon grape seed, coconut oil, licorice etc help eradicate microbes from the body and rebuild tissues by directly deactivating the microbial cells wall and replicating machinery by the action of the secondary compounds in plants that includes the alkaloids

Botanicals also indirectly shut off the infective ability of microbes by the following actions:

- By producing sterols and sterolins,they stop inflammation that act as fuel for microbial multiplication
- By the action of the anti oxidation system, they change our metabolism from fermentation to oxidation. When cells replace sugar with oxygen for its metabolic needs, microbes dye off.
- By removing wastes and toxins from the blood, herbal remedies increase its oxygen carrying capacities. Microbes cannot survive in an oxygen rich blood
- Herbs like cleavers and calendula help clean the lymphatic system of wastes that made the immune system sluggish. When we free the lymphatic system of wastes we restore the activities of the white blood cells and interferon that makes our internal environment uninhabitable to microbes
- Herbs like milk thistle and dandelion helpstrenfhten organ , restore liver function, makes the liver more able to make disease fighting nutrients and filter out wastes that slow down metabolism.

Examples

Goldenseal (Hydrastis canadensis) contains a high content of isoquinoline alkaloids, of which berberine is the most widely studied. Berberine has also been shown to activate macrophages. Berberine is generally non-toxic at recommended doses, but it is not recommended for use during pregnancy, and it can decrease B vitamin absorption. It may interfere with H-2 antagonists, proton pump inhibitors, antihypertensives, barbiturates and sedatives, and heparin.

Licorice root (Glychrrhiza glabra) has, as its major active component a triterpenoid saponin, glycyrrhizic acid. Intestinal flora hydrolyzes glycyrrhizin yielding the aglycone molecule (glycyrrhentinic acid) and a sugar moiety. Both glycyrrhizin and glycyrrhentinic acid have been shown to induce interferon. This leads to significant antiviral activity. Licorice root has been shown to directly inhibit the growth of several DNA and RNA viruses in cell cultures (vaccinia, herpes simplex, Newcastle disease, vesicular stomatitis virus) and to irreversibly inactivate HSV. The herb also shows antimicrobial activity in vitro against Staphylococcus aureus, Streptococcus mutans, Mycobacterium, and Candida albicans. Licorice compounds are showing promise in the treatment of HIV related diseases and chronic Hepatitis B. Other natural remedies with antimicrobial properties includes Oregon grape seed, bayberry, olive leaf and the coconut oil

From the foregoing, we can infer that that the alkaloids in plants are directly responsible for its antimicrobial properties. Indirect actions of plants include reduction of toxic loads in the tissues when we clean the blood and lymph. When we use a wide variety of herbs in an herbal tonic, the multiplication of their synergistic effects overwhelm infective agents like the HIV, hepatitis and other microbes that plague humanity. With this approach Dr Peter Oyakhire was able to change his hepatitis viral load from 'too numerous to count to undetectable'.

In 1994, 26 years later, independent researchers developed an extraction process that created a potent broad spectrum olive leaf extract that is currently commercially available.

The olive leaf extract derived from the olive leaf (Olean europea L) is a natural, non-toxic anti-microbial remedy. It is one of nature's most potent virucides. Oleuropein is present throughout the whole leaf. It gives the olive leaf its disease-resistant properties. It helps protect the tree against predators, bacteria, and insects. It is found to inhibit the growth of every virus, bacterium, fungus, yeast, and protozoa it was tested against. It is potent against the HBV virus, too. When we consume the olive leaf, we acquire these resistant and protective properties of the plant.

Medicinal Mushrooms Complex: Nature's Vaccine
Botanist classifies mushrooms as a fungus. Unlike plants which generate nutrients through photosynthesis, they get majority of their nutrients from dead organic matter or soil which makes them organic recyclers that convert dead decaying matter into nutrients. Mushrooms appear when the right nutrients are amassed under right environmental conditions. They release their spores into the wind at maturity, and they start the maturation cycle all over again when soil and environmental conditions are right. Like vaccines, mushrooms stimulate the immune system and inhibit tumor growth indirectly due to the presence of immune-activating polysaccharides which are repeating units of glucose molecules. These giant, complex, branched chain-like sugar molecules are similar to the ones found in the cell membranes of bacteria. Consequently, when we consume them, they "fool" or trick our immune system into believing that an actual infection is under way. Then the immune cells begin to roam the body chopping down bacteria, yeast, viruses, or tumor cells and mount immune responses while posing no threat. This response has been shown to activate the macrophages, interferon, and the killer cells that destroy invading pathogens.

Doctors Health advisory: I highly recommend a complex that includes reishi, coriolus, and lentinula edodes (LEM), an extract and powdered derivative from the mycelium of shiitake mushrooms before the cap and the stem matures, to provide abundance a supply of polysaccharides. The polysaccharides in mushrooms are often bound to various proteins that closely represent the unique identity of the organism and thus often activate the immune systems as they enter the body. These protein-bound polysaccharides in medicinal fungi can often lead to exaggerated immune responses that lead to a variety of allergic reactions.

Echinacea have immuno-stimulating and immuno-modulating properties that act by significantly increasing phagosytic activities of the immune surveillance system. Echinacea works by stimulating the white blood cells and bringing more white blood cells to the area of an infection faster by amplifying the distress signal sent out by attacked cells. It also increases the aggressiveness of white blood cells toward intruding pathogens. Unlike drugs that stimulate the immune system in a unidirectional manner, Echinacea is an immuno-tonic that has bi-directional characteristics. Daniel Mowrey, in his book *Herbal Tonic Therapies* indicates that immuno-tonics restore homeostatic balance to the immune system, regardless of which way the immune system deviates from normal, by sending two possible contradictory signals bi-directionally. Thus, if a person has a low white blood cell count, Echinacea can stimulate the immune system to produce more white blood cells. Conversely, in individuals with an elevated white blood count, Echinacea can help decelerate the production of white blood cells. Echinacea has a strong activating influence on the body's macrophage-mediated defense system which destroys cancerous cells and pathogens.

Doctor's Health Advisory.
Echinacea should be used cautiously in people allergic to plants of the sunflower family or ragweed. Since it stimulates the immune system, it should not be used for extended periods of time by people with auto immune diseases.

Chapter 8

Healing (Get Well) Crises

Transitioning from Illness to Wellness

A healing crisis is the result of the body working to eliminate waste products through all elimination channels and to set the stage for regeneration. The end result: old tissues are replaced with new ones. When any treatment or cleansing program causes a large scale die-off of microbes, a significant amount of wastes are released into the body. The more microbes present, and the stronger their endotoxins, the stronger the cleansing reaction. When any treatment or de-tox causes the organs of the body to release their stored poisons and toxins, particularly the liver, which is a storehouse of drug and poison residues, a cleansing reaction usually take place. Any program, such as fasting, which causes a rapid deterioration of fat cells (which are a storehouse for toxins), can cause a get-well crisis as toxins previously lodged in the fat cells are released.

One crisis is not always enough for a complete cure. The person in a chronic "locked" disease state will often have to go through cycles of healing crises, with each one improving the condition some. It has taken time to develop a chronically-diseased state, and time is required to let go of the "locked" energy, piece by piece. It's like peeling the layers off an onion. With a more serious condition, there may be many small crises to go through before the system can become healthily balanced.

The Philosophy of Get-Well Crises

This philosophy of natural healing requires crises to occur before true healing can take place. This is anti-ethical to orthodox approaches to healing that have a drug for every crisis. In mainstream medicine, it is assumed that a patient who is free of disease symptoms is more or less healthy. The aim of drugs is to achieve this condition by removing disagreeable symptoms.

The philosophy of the get-well crises is likened to "Herring's Law of Cure", which states that *"All cure starts from within out, from the head down and in reverse order as the symptoms have appeared."* Dr. John Whitman Ray has developed a method specifically designed to help us travel the long road to superior health. He calls it *body electronics*, using nutrition as well as press point therapy to facilitate emotional release and expansion of consciousness. Out of this work Dr. Ray found it necessary to modify Herring's Law to the following:

LAW OF HEALING CRISIS
A get-well crisis will occur only when an individual is ready both mentally and physically. A get-well crisis will begin from inside out, in opposite order, chronologically, as to how the symptoms appeared and commensurate with the severity of the trauma. The individual will have the opportunity to re-experience each trauma— physiological and psychological— beginning with the trauma of least severity. It must be recognised that traumas involving emotions, which include all traumas, will be released in order, beginning with unconsciousness, then apathy, grief, fear, anger, pain, and eventually enthusiasm (love), in conjunction with the appropriate words for each emotion and thought pattern (sensory memory) which are accessible at each level. Unconditional love and unconditional forgiveness are the keys to applying and transmuting resistance at any level, once these resistances are brought to view through the application of the laws of love, light, and perfection.

With this definition Dr. Ray emphasises the importance of the psychosomatic side of our health problems. Each disease, accident, or surgical intervention contains a strong emotional component which needs to be re-experienced during a reaction, otherwise the healing will remain incomplete and the problem will present itself again at a later time for healing at a deeper level. This also means that the body selects the kind of healing crisis that is most appropriate at the time, taking into consideration its needs and abilities to have a certain area healed or improved. We can consciously influence this choice by working on a particular problem. The body also tries to select a perfect timing, which does not disable us during important events coming up. We are guided on our healing path by our inner intelligence, which has our best interest at heart, and which chooses the best time to express a get well crisis. In the beginning, our healing reactions will be mainly on the physical or biological level, but, more and more, we will experience the release of emotional blocks and changes in consciousness, preparing us for greater activity on the spiritual level.

"What we sow or plant in the soil will come back to us in exact kind, but we entirely disregard this law when it comes to mental sowing." Orison Swett Marden

The body has an innate desire for normal health. We have the capacity to earn our way back to normal health no matter how bad our current situation is that state, no matter how "normal" or bad our health is now. But, to get from illness to wellness the body must go through a transition process referred to as an elimination phase of healing. This elimination process is often referred to as the "healing crisis" or the "get-well crisis." This is primarily a cleansing reaction like the discomfort encountered when using an antiseptic to fumigate the house. While the fumigation process may be uncomfortable, the ensuring cleanliness is otherwise rewarding. Once the healing crisis starts, reactions may be mild or severe. Expect ups and downs as it takes awhile to get good health back.

Studies show that when patients engage in some manner of systemic waste removal one of the first manifestations exhibited is a revisiting of the same symptoms formerly present when a patient had a specific ailment in the past. Also known as the "Herxheimer Reaction", this reaction occurs when the body tries to eliminate toxins at a faster rate than they can be properly disposed of. The more toxic and sick we are, the more severe the get-well or healing crisis. It is characterized by a temporary increase in symptoms during the cleansing or de-tox process which may be mild or severe. You may feel worse and therefore conclude that the treatment is not working. But, these reactions are signs that the treatment is working and that your body is going through the process of cleaning itself of impurities, toxins, and imbalances.

During a *disease crisis*, the body usually has great difficulty expelling toxic waste. The accumulation of this morbid matter throughout the body leads from acute to sub-acute tissue inflammation. If the condition is left unchecked, the sub-acute symptoms can deteriorate to chronic or degenerative disease. During the disease-reversal process that eventually results in a *healing crisis*, the body experiences many of the same symptoms present during a disease crisis. These symptoms generally last no longer than a few days, and all of the body's channels of waste elimination work very hard to expel toxic waste, particularly fecal matter, urine, and catarrh. Sometimes, discomfort during the healing crisis is of greater intensity than when you were developing the chronic disease. This may explain why there may be a brief flare-up in one's condition. Often, the crisis will come after you feel your very best. Most people feel somewhat ill during the first few days of a cleanse because it is at that point that your body dumps toxins into the blood stream for elimination. With a more serious condition, there may be many small crises to go through before the final one occurs. In any case, a cleansing and purifying process is underway, and stored wastes are in a free-flowing state.

Healing crises are made fifty times worse in enzyme-deficient individual. Avoid carbonated drinks and fluoridated or chlorinated water during detoxification and healing crises because they destroy enzymes. Carbonated drinks are high in phosphorus that leaches needed calcium out of the body. The digestion of meat uses lots of calcium, minerals, and enzymest. Other substances that hinder enzymes are antibiotics taken for illness, any food treated with pesticides, any animal given antibiotics, and alcohol. Individuals who have had radiation or chemotherapy, are low in enzymes, too, and require lots of natural supplementation with enzymes.

How do I Differentiate between Healing crises and Actual Disease Crises?

The famous nutritionist Dr. Bernard Jensen lists these ways to differentiate between healing crises and an actual diseases crisis:

- A healing crisis is accompanied by elimination, as the body is actively releasing wastes that include chemicals and drugs, which manifests as acute conditions of the underlining illness.
- Organ breakdown and dysfunction are not accompanied by increased elimination of wastes.
- Before and during healing crises, eliminative channels work well as they respond to the exit of wastes from the body. In disease crises, elimination does not work well before the crises and may worsen or stop during the crises.

- During healing crises, stored mucous, catarrh, and other wastes become less solid as they are thrown out of the body during purification. In disease crises, catarrh is not eliminated and mucus is old, thick, chronic, and congestive.

When do Healing Crises Occur?

Healing crises often come suddenly when we think we have overcome our health issues. They manifest themselves after the old tissues have been exchanged with the newer ones and there is enough energy to complete the exchange and elimination of the old tissues. They come on when the body has sufficient strength to violently rid itself of the old wastes, says Dr. Jensen. He indicates that organ regeneration passes through three phases, namely, elimination, transition, and re-building. The healing crisis occurs at the end of the transitional stage when the new tissues have matured enough to take on the function of a more healthy body.

Healing crises also occur during fasting, use of antibiotic herbs, chelating agents, juicing, and any detoxification program. The separation and eliminations of toxins ultimately establishes new standards for our homeostasis. Our body's resistance to this change is evidenced by Herxheimer reactions. This is a time when the body is doing its housecleaning of impurities and toxins as it approach homeostasis. The body is releasing accumulated toxins that have been stored in the body for a long time, probably since childhood. The body is also releasing more toxins than it can handle through the blood stream and its eliminative channels. Individuals with stronger constitutions experience fewer crises while those with weaker constitutions experience more. The more toxic an individual is, the more severe the crises. Orthodox practitioners suppress these crises with drugs, while alternative practitioners depend upon and look for them as the astrologer looks at the stars. Conventional suppression of healing crises makes the ordinary experience of life a diagnosis which makes patients out of healthy people. Like going through the dark nights of the soul, the following symptoms can be expected:
- temporary exacerbation of the disease symptoms that may be identical to the disease itself
- worse feelings that make one feel that the remedy is not working, whereas they indicate that the treatment is actually working
- healing reactions that last from a few days to several weeks

- a discomfort discovered during healing crises that is greater than the chronic diseases itself, depending on the level of individual toxicity

What causes healing crises?

It is caused by the body eliminating toxins from its tissues to prepare the ground for regeneration. Scripturally, you cannot pour new wine into old wine skins. In infectious diseases, it is due to die-offs of bacteria or viruses releasing their endotoxins. The more infected an individual is, the more potent are the endotoxins released into the blood stream for the eliminative channels to handle. This is why a lot of emphasis is placed on opening up the eliminative channels during detoxification. The liver is a store house for the majority of what we ingest. Any de-tox program, like fasting, often leads to the rapid release of stored toxins from the fat tissues and this often leads to healing crises.

What are common symptoms of healing crises?

Body odor and bad breath from the release of poisonous gas and, toxins, diarrhea, cramps, headaches, aches, pains, fatigue, nausea, fever, sinus congestion, skin eruptions, disorientation, sleepiness, shooting pains, muzziness in the head area, dizziness, anxiety, and strong emotions of anger, anxiety, sadness, fear, and depression. Mood swings and suppressed memories arise, too.

How are healing crises addressed?

When healing crises are experienced, it is best to work with an experienced herbalist or alternative healthcare practitioner who can offer assurance and guidance.

- Activate the eliminative channels.
- Drink plenty of fluids, water, and herbal teas to flush the toxins out of the body, preferably 4 – 6 glasses of water daily.
- It is important to follow the healing crises with enemas or colonics to help eliminate toxins.
- Reduction of dosage and/or cessation is recommended
- Massage therapy, acupuncture, and rest help facilitate the process.
- The temptation to take a pain reliever or other such remedies to stop the symptoms defeats the whole purpose of the cleansing and increases the toxic load. It shuts the process

down. When this happens, the garbage remains and builds up more firepower to do us harm.

- If pain is too severe, it is recommended to take an analgesic.

After the healing crises, what next?

- Make sure the vacuum created is not filled with old pattern of behaviors. Remember in the Bible when Jesus cast out demons. He warned the people to fill their life with righteousness or else the demons would come back seven times greater to repossess the body.
- It is important to cultivate healthy patterns of living and thinking that befits the exercise.

Chapter 9

Is the Immune System the Lymphatic System?

In all the medical jargon you have read about the immune system, it is important to realize that the immune system is the lymphatic system's compartment. The immune system is a system nature put into place to shield humans from extreme conditions and imbalances in the environment. The activities of the immune system are fully integrated with the lymphatic system. White blood cells reside in the lymphatic system, and when we optimize the activities of the lymphatic system with efficient management of the cellular wastes it collects, we are said to have an efficient immune system. It works efficiently when there is physiological continuity of its performance with other systems in the body. It receives metabolic wastes, and filters and neutralizes harmful agents and microbes before returning them to systemic circulation. Individuals who have properly-functioning lymphatic systems have good immune systems, and those who have sluggish lymphatic systems have weak immune systems which are predisposed to cancer and organ degenerations. The immune system is said to be weak when we are unable to eliminate cellular metabolic wastes and neutralize pathogens. Immune system activities take place in the lymphatic system. The immune system evolved because we have lived side by side with microbes and external environments that can often times threaten our existence. Our technological advances accelerate much faster than the human body can catch up with them. Our cellular metabolism is not designed to handle our current diet, lifestyles, and environmental pressures. As we begin to incorporate botanicals into our daily menu, we aid the immune system in doing its work with the different components of our bodily systems.

The ancients believe that the human body is like an irrigation system that is traversed by three great rivers that cleanse and maintains the body's systems. These are the white river or the lymphatic system, the red river or the cardiovascular system, and the brown river or the digestive system. The overall health of an individual and freedom from chronic degenerative disease is contingent on the integrity of these rivers. As we journey to explore these forgotten rivers of health, reversal of all chronic degenerations becomes inevitable. We observe how pets stretch their bodies after waking up. Animals are constantly on the move in their habitats, and fishes are constantly mobile in their water environment. It is only flowing streams that native peoples use for domestic activities. When the body stretches, muscles are contracted. The weakening of the body is not due to the effects of illness, but to the neglect of its metabolism resulting from the accumulation of toxins from stagnation. Removal of toxins from cells and intercellular spaces is a process requiring constant stimulation of cells by nerve impulses, which occurs during exercise or movement, which causes contractions of muscles. When people do not exercise or move efficiently, such as is done in stretching, aerobics, running, walking, and dancing, their bodies gradually decline and degenerate.

Dr. Reckeweg, M.D., the father of homotoxicology

According to Dr. Reckeweg, M.D., the father of homotoxicology, "As long as the body eliminates toxic wastes, the body maintains health, even if health is at an extreme illness level." This emphasizes the significance of re-establishing the flow of interstitial fluid within the organs' intercellular structure to sustain health. This proves that the endothelial gap's malfunction is the culprit the development of "disease" states. When mechanical dysfunction is rectified, treatment is one step closer to advancing toward success in disease management." He points out that when the lymph system malfunctions, excess toxins and large proteins accumulate within the intercellular spaces, causing inflammation. When the fluid pressure in the intercellular space is high (too much fluid), the endothelial gaps are impaired in their function. Our metabolic waste products include diacetic, lactic, pyruvic, uric, carbonic, acetic, butyric, and hepatic acids. The staging, type, or location of classification of your disease is irrelevant to its cause and cure as long as we remove impediments to cure.

If toxic wastes are not removed by the lymphatic system, they cause organ degeneration of the weakest or the most venerable body parts and death. Intercellular fluid accumulates on the outside of the endothelial gap, and inflammation and degeneration occurs. In diseased conditions, the intercellular spaces between cells are wet and flooded with proteinous cellular wastes, like a blockage and backup in the home plumbing system. This process is similar to what happens in a swimming pool during a heavy rainstorm. When too much water is trying to get through the flap covering the drain on the side of the pool, the flap closes and water cannot drain from the pool. The water level rises, reaches the brim, and spills out, carrying debris into the surrounding area. When the endothelial gap is processing, fluid in the intercellular space maintains the cells "dry state" level, and intercellular space is free of toxins and disease. The theme of this book is to educate you on how to activate the lymphatic – immune system and reverse your chronic degenerative diseases.

Dr. Alfred Pischinger and the regulation of the extracellular matrix

Dr. Alfred Pischinger was the first scientist to develop a theory for complementary or holistic medicine based on the regulation of the extracellular matrix (ground regulation). He was born in Linz, Austria in 1899 and died in 1983 in Graz. In his book Dr Pischinger stated that the extracellular space is responsible for all of the basic vital functions: providing nutrition, waste removal, acid – alkaline balance, and cell communication, as well as aiding in inflammatory and immune processes. Long overlooked, the proper regulation of the extracellular space is the key to successfully treating all infections, cancer, diabetes, and other chronic degenerative diseases. While orthodox medicine relies mainly on the cells and their biochemistry, often overlooked are the extracellular fluids or matrix in which cells are embedded as being pivotal to health. This "matrix" or ground regulation system, as Dr. Pischinger called it, supports, nurtures, and detoxifies all cells and tissues by supplying them with critically-needed nutrients such as oxygen, hormone messengers, and by removing cellular waste products, toxins, and other residues so that health can be restored and immunity enhanced.

In this day and age, it is easy to become over-burdened with toxins and metabolic wastes—and it is not always our fault. Every year, hundreds of thousands of new chemicals are released on the market, many not fully tested for their effects on the human body. Different toxins, such as chemicals, heavy metals, viruses, bacterial residues, indoor pollutants, diet, metabolic wastes, antibiotics, and other drugs remains are stored in the extracellular space where they cause stagnation and harm to the cells. Given enough time, these toxins exceed the storage capacity of the ECM and impair the ability of the body to regulate and regenerate, causing rapid non-specific symptoms to emerge, e.g. fatigue, headache, muscular pain, mood swings, and allergies. Our immune – lymphatic system shuts down. It can no longer compensate for the toxic overload within us, and it leaves us a sitting duck for all kinds of viruses, bacteria, chronic degenerative diseases, and other microbes to move in. The viscous cycle continues as your now-toxic body is actually turned into a playground for these unwanted guests that are having the time of their life at our expense.

Lymphology and the immune system

The American Association of Lymphology indicates that laboratory research and studies on the cause and cure of all diseases were done between 1930 and 1963 at the Harvard, Tulane, and the University of Mississippi medical schools by Doctors Cecil H Drinker, H. S Myerson, and Arthur C. Guyton, but were suppressed by special interest groups. They believe that every healing art involves the movement of oxygen into the cells, while all illness, including cancer, involves the movement of oxygen away from the cells. According to Dr. C. Samuel West, blood proteins and water must be removed from the spaces between the cells, referred to as intercellular space, by the lymphatic vessels to keep the cells in what is called the "healthy dry state." In this situation, the cells effectively burn complex carbohydrates to produce carbon dioxide, water, and energy. If this does not happen, the blood proteins and water around the cells will alter the "dry state" to the "diseased wet state." This produces a lack of oxygen and loss of energy at the cell level, which is the cause of all diseases that afflict humanity. If there is insufficient oxygen at the cellular level, the metabolism will be incomplete, and carbon dioxide and lactic acid will be produced. Carbon dioxide displaces oxygen from the hemoglobin and prevents the red blood cells from getting the needed oxygen for cellular functions.

Organs near the stagnation point are awash in their own wastes, cannot take in nutrients, and cannot eliminate wastes. Studies show that excess blood proteins and water leave the blood stream under conditions of shock, stress, toxicity, malnutrition or injury. Healing occurs when we pull out all of the dead cells, poisons, excess blood proteins, and water from around the cells to keep them in what is called the "dry state" so they can get the oxygen they need. The diseased "wet state" constitutes a shift from oxidation to fermentation. In this condition, the rate of production of diseased cells outweighs their rate of destruction. Oxygen oxidizes or mop up toxic waste build up. Its deficiency is the culprit in all diseases; it creates a state of cellular confusion or drowning. It occurs when the human body's oxygen availability, demand, and utilization drops lower than normal due to exposure to conditions that stems from malnutrition, environmental pollution, physical inactivity, stress, and westernization of ancestral life. These conditions suffocate our cells because the supply of oxygen falls short of our demand; metabolism is faulty, immunity is lowered, and the cells shift from using oxygen (an aerobic process) for metabolism to predominately using sugar (an anaerobic process). Herein lies the etiology of all diseases.

We are all a step away from disease. If you are dealing with chronic degenerative diseases, total eradication of symptoms is not the ultimate goal. Effective management and repair of the metabolic pathways with nutrition and lifestyles changes are a lifetime commitment with the aim of being a step ahead of the game.

A general understanding of the lymphatic system will buttress the need for lymphatic massage, deep breathing, and physical exercise for detoxification. It plays a crucial role in the body's ability to ward off illnesses and recover from diseases. The lymphatic system is twice the size of the circulatory system. Like the cardiovascular system, movement is key to its optimal function, and sluggishness leads to their failure. Like a house with two plumbing systems, one different from the other in having a one-way valve filtration system and the other having a central pump, the lymphatic system runs parallel to the vascular system. While the cardiovascular system supplies blood and nutrients to the tissues, the lymphatic system runs side by side with the vascular system to collect the leftover intracellular wastes for purification, filtration, and recycling. Nature put this in place to offset the danger of tissue wastes hanging around the body. It is often referred to as the body's sewage-disposal system.

Understanding the Immune System: The Key to Healing Liver Disease

193

A good understanding of the immune system and use of aggressive natural remedies can replace all of the damaged liver cells within an eighteen-month period, since the life span of each liver cell is about eighteen months.

The body's immune defense has more influence in determining the progression of chronic hepatitis to cirrhosis than remedies and drugs that exclusively address the viral loads. The immune system can be modulated in cases of individual illnesses, which helps in understanding the root of immune deficiencies and points to potential avenues that. The immune system has many weapons in its responses against viral assault on our body. The immune systems use specialized proteins build from amino acids that are derived from food. The two main fluid systems in the body are the blood and the lymph. Immune enhancement is the foundation upon which all alternative remedies are built; the immune system is basically the lymphatic system, and its various components that include the white blood cells and the lymph nodes.

All blood cells are manufactured by stem cells, which reside mainly in the bone marrow via a process called hematopoiesis. The stem cells produce hemocytoblasts that differentiate into the precursors for all different types of blood cells namely, erythrocytes (red blood cells), thrombocytes (platelets), and leucocytes (white blood cells).

The leucocytes (white blood cells) are further subdivided into the granulocytes and the agranulocytes (no granules). The granulocytes are white blood cells that contain granules filled with potent chemicals that allow them to destroy the enemy. They contain the neutrophils, eosinophils, and basophiles. Neutrophils are one type of phagocyte. It uses its pre-packaged chemicals to ingest microbes. Eosinophils and basophiles de-regranulate by spraying into microbes. Eosinophiles congregate at the sites of allergic and parasitic reactions. They release enzymes to relieve the biochemical causes of allergic attacks.

The agranulocytes are the lymphocytes (B-cells and T-cells), and the monocytes. The lymphocytes circulate in the blood and in the lymph system, and make their home in the lymphoid organs. The primary lymphoid organs are the bone marrow and the thymus gland, which is located behind the breast bone above the heart. The secondary lymphoid organs are located at or near any possible port of entry of pathogens. They are found in the adenoids, tonsils, spleen (at upper left of the abdomen), lymph nodes (that dot the lymphatic vessels in the neck, armpits, abdomen, and groin), Peyer's patch within the intestines, and in the appendix. Although not considered a lymphatic organ, the liver produces the majority of the body's lymph.

Both the T-cells and B-cells originate in the bone marrow. When the T-cells mature, they are instructed in their duties in the thymus gland. The T stands for thymus. The B cells mature in the bone marrow; the B stands for bone marrow.

The size of the thymus gland diminishes with age and this necessitates the need for thymus extract in the treatment of immune deficiency diseases.
Approximately, one sixth of the entire body consists of the space between cells called the interstitium. The fluid within this space is called the interstitial fluid. This fluid flows into the lymphatic vessels and becomes the lymph. The lymph vessels, like veins, have one-way valves that prevent back flow. Along these vessels are small bean-shaped lymph nodes that serve as filters of the lymphatic vessels.

Types of immunity
Humans have three types of immunity against diseases, namely, innate, adaptive, and passive.
- *Innate immunity* is what we are born with, and it is non-specific. This is our first line of defense in preventing diseases. All antigens are attacked pretty much equally. It is genetically based, and we pass it on to our offering. Innate immunity also includes the external barriers of the body, like the skin and mucous membranes that line the nose, throat, and the gastrointestinal tract.
- *Adaptive immunity* involves the lymphocytes, and develops as children and adults are exposed to diseases or immunized against diseases through vaccination. Passive immunity is borrowed from another source, and last for a short time e.g. antibodies in mother's milk.

The immune system is characterized by the following.
- *Antigen-specific* It recognizes and acts against particular antigens. A foreign substance that invades the body and elicits an immune response is called an antigen.

- *Systemic* It is not confined to the initial site but works throughout the body.
- *Memory* It recognizes and mounts an even stronger attack to the same antigen next time

Disorders of the immune system can be broken down into four main categories:
- immunodeficiency disorders (primary or acquired),e.g. the AIDS epidemic
- autoimmune disorders (the body's own immune system turns on itself as foreign matter), e.g. lupus, scleroderma, autoimmune hepatitis, and sarcoid
- Allergic disorders (immune system overreacts in response to a foreign matter referred to as an allergen), e.g. asthma, eczema, and hay fever.
- cancers of the immune systems, e.g. lymphoma and leukemia

Antibodies ambush antigens in the body fluids. The job of attacking the antigens is left to the other components of the immune system, mainly the lymphocytes, via two main systems, cell-mediated and humoral. The cell-mediated or Th1 system refers to immune mechanisms not controlled or mediated by antibodies. This involves white blood cells called the T cells (thymus dependent) and other specialized immune cells. They are non-specific primary agents of the immune systems. They also patrol the blood and the lymph. T cells contribute to the immune system in two major ways: They direct and regulate the immune response. Others kill infected or cancerous human cells. The humoral (Th2) or antibody-mediated systems depend on the B cells (bone-marrow dependent). This is called humoral immunity because the antibodies circulate in the blood and the lymph, which the ancient Greeks called the body's "humors." They are specific or secondary immune systems that originate in the bone marrow. They do not depend on the thymus gland.

Chapter 10

Detoxification and Liver Waste Management

*"Most people who eat standard American "goo and glue" diets have about 5 –
10 pounds of fecal matter stored in the colon. It is said that, according to the
autopsy, John Wayne had 40 pounds of impacted fecal matter in his body at
death. Elvis reportedly had 60 pounds."*
USA today, January, 11th 1999

What is Detoxification?

Detoxification is a metabolic process in which toxins are transformed into
less toxic, body-friendly, or more-readily excretal substances. If toxins
are not eliminated from the body, the eliminative organs are under the
influence of active toxins that are retained in the tissues where they hamper
organ functions all the way down to the cellular level. When toxins take
over an organ's functions, degenerative disease sets in. This ultimately calls
for detoxification and elimination.

Detoxification decreases toxic stresses which cause a sluggish liver.
Detoxification is the first step to restore immune system. To optimize the
performance of herbs, it is best to detoxify. Detoxification helps raise energy
levels, eradicates pathogens, stimulates bile production, stimulates blood
and lymphatic flow, promote mucus discharge from the lungs, hydrates
the colon, stimulates urine output, provides nutritional support for organs,
stimulates peristalsis, increases digestive capability and bowel function,
restores the body's ability to heal itself, and help facilitate absorption of
nutrients.

There are two forms of detoxification namely - internal and external.
Internal detoxification is the intake of botanical remedies through the
mouth or the anus. From the mouth, they pass through the digestive

system and are absorbed into the blood and lymph where they pull toxins from the tissues. The toxins are then returned to the kidneys and the intestines where they are eliminated as wastes. Colon hydrotherapy is a form of internal detoxification where water and/or botanical supplements are passed into the body from the rectum. Because they are not degraded by the stomach acids, they are more potent than orals. External detoxification involves the use of saunas, ionic foot detox, detox baths and massage therapy to pull toxins from the outside. When aggressive detoxification is required, both internal and external detoxification may be employed. However, for maintenance of health, oral detoxification may be combined with the external detoxification quaterly.The most commonly used herbs for oral detoxification are Burdock, Licorice, Dandelion, Yellow duck, Oregon grape root, and Tumeric,Paud Arco, Plantain leaves, Echinacea, Cleavers, Artichoke and Milk thistle. These herbs will heal the body, restore liver functions, create an environment unfavorable for viruses, flush the gallbladder, rebuild the liver and nourish the organ systems

By removing toxins from tissues and fat stores, it makes it easier for fats to burn as energy for cellular regeneration (Watson, 2006). Emotional toxins make the body produce excess stress, via hormones like adrenalin and cortisone which are stored in the liver. When these hormones stay too long in the liver, they cause degenerative diseases and immune dysfunctions. When detoxification is influenced with herbs and attitudinal changes, stored energy in the liver and in fats is activated and pathogens die-off. These manifest as healing (Herxheirmer) reactions that include toxic headaches, flu-like symptoms, sluggishness, mood swings, sensitivities, allergic reactions, die-off of pathogens, and symptoms that mimic the initial disease. These symptoms, when suppressed with drugs, stop the healing process. If allowed to run their course under the care of an experienced naturopath, they are usually followed by feelings of euphoria and wellness.

☒ *Flashback Detoxifications with colonics saved my life. It helped eliminate the effects of chemotherapy, prescription drugs, and lifelong accumulated toxins from my liver. It gave me a new lease on life. It help jumpstart my immune system as over 75 percent of the immunes system is located in the gut.*

According to the Environmental Protection Agency, in the year 2000 alone, more than 4 billion pounds of chemicals were released into the ground, over 260 million pounds of chemicals were discharged into the surface waters like lakes and rivers, and more than 2 billion pounds of chemical emissions were pumped into the air we breathe. With a total of over 6 billion pounds of chemical pollutants threatening our existence and physical health, we have an urgent need to detoxify. To compound the problem of our toxic environment, we have refined nutritional values out of the food we eat and added preservatives, antibiotics, colorings, and drugs to our menus.

How Much Toxin Are YOU Exposed to Daily?
- An average person walks around with about 25 pounds of toxic waste caked in the colon. (Brooner Jr., 2000)
- About 30,000 pounds of new toxins are added yearly to food, water, soil, and the environment. These all constitute internal pollution and put the liver in a precarious position when dealing with infections.
- Over 10,000 chemical solvents, emulsifiers, and preservatives are used in food processing and storage. (Cobb, 2004)
- Every week, approximately 6,000 new chemicals are listed in the chemical society journals, which add up to the 300,000 each year. (Lipski, 2000)
- An average of 14 pounds of preservatives, colorings, food additives, emulsifiers, flavorings, antimicrobials, and humectants are consumed yearly by each person. (Lipski, 2000)
- In 1990, the EPA estimated that there were about 70,000 chemicals used in pesticides, foods, and drugs. (Lipski, 2000)

How do Toxins Affect the Liver?
Toxicity has had a greater impact on the quality of life of mankind in this century than ever before because there are many more potent chemicals being produced. Toxicity occurs externally and internally—externally from the environment through breathing, ingestion, and physical contact, and internally from toxins generated as our body synthesizes what we put in our bodies.

"The doctor of the future will give no medicine but will interest his patients in the care of the human frame, diet and the cause and prevention of disease" and not the symptoms"
Thomas Edison

Stresses associated with excessive toxins from the food, water, and environment makes the liver sluggish. The liver, the digestive system, and the immune system are so intricately linked that it is impossible to remedy hepatitis and liver disease without an emphasis on digestive health. Degenerative diseases like hepatitis are often associated with a toxic sluggish liver, stagnation, gallstones, and blockage of the bile ducts. This necessitates the need for an aspect of detoxifications that facilitates opening the exit channels and cleansing the toxins from the body to avoid them being reabsorbed back into the body.

Environmental toxins enter the body through the skin and the lungs, and find their way into systemic circulation which passes them to the liver for detoxification. Similarly, improperly digested foods are acted upon by the unfriendly bacteria in the colon. This makes for the multiplication of these harmful bacteria beyond the population of the beneficial bacteria. When this happens, putrefaction occurs as rotten food produces chemical toxins that irritate the linings of the colon and lets toxins leak into the body through the gut. These toxins also pass through the portal veins and go directly to the liver, carrying food, nutrients toxins, nitrogen, and fluids from the colon to the liver. (Tipps, 2002, Watson, 2006 and Gilbere, 2004)

The liver does the following with toxins: (Brooner Jr., 2000)
- It burns them up during the metabolic process like food.
- It eliminates them through the eliminative channels.
- It binds them for storage in the cells and tissues where they disrupt cellular functions and cause organ degeneration.

How do Toxins Cause Organ Degeneration?
Studies show that about 90 percent of all metabolic activities in the cells take place in the cell membranes. Toxins inculcate themselves in the cell membranes, displace nutrients, and disrupt metabolic activities. The liver becomes swollen and puts pressure on adjourning organs which results in pain. Most drugs, like toxins, are mostly lipid-soluble. When taken, they have to be processed by the liver before being absorbed and used by the body. Water-soluble drugs are not well absorbed by the body and have difficulty getting to the bloodstream. When these toxins overburden the liver, they hamper its functions, and the liver becomes sluggish and overflows through the hepatic veins into systemic circulation. They make the liver

cells porous, exacerbates free-radical damage, and cause viral infections to become infective. From systemic circulation, these toxins are deposited in the organs and tissues of the body. They interfere with metabolism at the cellular level and result in constitutional acidity. Toxins are stored in fat tissues where they fuel irritations and chronic inflammations that lead to progressive degenerative liver diseases. They are trapped in the fat cells and cell membranes where they influence cellular functions. They are not easily eliminated from the human body. The discomforts associated with these occurrences manifest as signs and symptoms which orthodox medicine addresses with suppressive drugs. Through a series of biofeedback mechanisms, the body builds its homeostasis around these drugs that establishes a "pacifier effect." For optimal health, the human body requires an 80: 20 alkaline-to-acid ratio. Over 96 percent of prescription and non-prescription drugs are toxic and create acid-forming reactions in the body (Anderson, 2004. Baroody, 2002). Viruses and organ degeneration thrive best under acidic conditions. This approach marks the end of health care for the patient and the beginning of disease care by the doctor, making disease care the fastest growing failing enterprise in the world (Holford, 1999).

Like all filters, the liver's pores become clogged with toxins which disrupt its filtration ability. Consequently, contaminants that cannot be filtered are stored in the liver, which in turn creates pressure build-up within the liver. The ability to filter out new contaminants is also hampered. This leads to back-ups, and the toxin that cannot be filtered circulates in the body and the different organs and tissues in the body at cellular level. The storage of these accumulated lipid-soluble toxins in the membranes of the liver cells increases the workload of the immune system and degenerative diseases emerge. If the filtration pores are clogged, the liver is enlarged and immunological functions are jeopardized. This ultimately calls for detoxification.

How do herbs differ from vegetables and fruit juices in healing the body of diseases?

Fruits and vegetables primarily supply the body with deficient nutrients and the body utilize them to rebuild its defenses against diseases .Herbs work like a 'two edged sword'. They resupply nutritional deficiencies and concurrently have more potent phytonutrients or secondary compounds which actually go and fight disease cells, viruses and rebuild the body.

Ironically herbs are more superior to fruits and vegetable juices when dealing with healing. Because of their proximity to the minerals in the soil, root herbs are more potent than leaves, fruits and flowers. After the roots, nutrients move upwards against gravity and diminishing efficacy towards the stem, the bark, and the branches before we have flowers, leaves and fruits which are used for the juices. However, through the action of photosynthesis assorted colors of fruits, vegetables and leaves serves as a rich source of nutrients for our healing. It is advisable to combine both of them for optimal healing. Botanical remedies have complex intelligence system that go counter to the intelligence of disease cells. These complex systems utilize a process called 'Phyto confusion' to confuse and overwhelm disease cells to influence healing. The phyto confusion theory is propagated for the first time by Dr Peter Oyakhire

Detoxification and Healing with Green Drinks

Detoxification done with vegetable and fruit juices (or powdered super foods) supplies enzymes for the detoxification process, replenish pro-biotics after colonics, pull toxins from cells and tissues, binds heavy metals from the blood, tissues, and organs, while nourishing the body with the deficient essential nutrients and immunological building blocks (Page, 1999). Fruits and vegetables are some of the surest ways to deliver nutrients, antioxidants, anti-inflammatory agents, and pro-biotics from the soil. They also deliver oxygen directly to the human body, since most filtered, purified, distilled, and tap water is devoid of nutrients. Organic fruits and vegetables bring the human body closer to what nature intended. The enzymatic component of fruits and vegetable juices strips cancer cells of their incentives to metastasize. They create the greatest opportunity where enzymes and co-enzymes (vitamins) can come into the body together and work together to influence constitutional alkalinity and metabolic harmony. They have strong properties that can reach deep into the cells, tissues, and organs, and pull and neutralize toxins through a chelating process. Detoxification is similar to any external cleansing regimen that requires water and solvents. The water takes the solvents to places where cleansing is needed and then carries the dirt away. The solvents dissolve the dirt and make it easier for the water to flush it away. In humans, the solvents are the herbal remedies and vegetable juices that have the ability to pull, attract, and dissolve toxins through a chelating process (Koyfman, 2001).

Taking Care of the Digestive Tract

The bowels are where most toxins find their way into general body tissues through enterohepatic circulation. We cannot start the organ-rebuilding process without cleaning the bowels of accumulated caked fecal matter. As Gloria Gilbere puts it *"If the gut is not healthy, neither is the rest of the body."*

In the digestive tract, when food does not pass quickly, the proteins turn putrid and rot, fats become rancid, and carbohydrates ferment. The importance of periodic enemas or colonics is predicated on the fact that humans are instinctively cultured to clean their exteriors (that includes hairs, teeth, nails and body) regularly but to neglect their interiors. When the colon is cleaned the liver, pancreas, and gallbladder are relived of a lot of toxins.

Surgeons and gastroenterologists do not impress the significance of hardened fecal matter on their patients because they are not trained to know the consequences of these mucoid plaques. Until they mix with fecal matter, they are indistinguishable from that of a healthy person during endoscopy.

Why is Fiber Significant?

Consumption of fiber-rich foods will decrease the ability of the released bile and other intestinal toxins during detoxifications from being reabsorbed (auto intoxication) into the liver. Fiber adds bulk to waste, helps retain water in the colon which promotes softer and larger stool, expands in the colon, stimulates peristalsis in the colon, and binds to toxins that build up on the intestinal walls, pulling them along. This ultimately reduces the transit time and facilitates the movement of waste. Fiber scrubs the intestinal walls like a sponge and carries with it the toxins dumped in there during detoxification for excretion through the rectum. Ultimately, this reduces the availability and production of nitrogenous waste in the colon. Fiber also binds noxious bile acids, endotoxins, and bacteria products in the digestive tract. It provides substances for the bowel muscles to work on (Jensen, 1981). Fiber helps lower blood cholesterol, reduces the risk of colon and rectal cancer, and reduces bowel-transit time. Dietary sources of fiber are flax seeds, whole grains, cereals, legumes, fruits, bran, and cruciferous vegetables that are raw or lightly steamed.

What is an Enema?

The colon has always been referred to as the second brain since almost all of the operational centers of the immune system reside in the digestive tract. Nutritionists and naturopaths believe that life begins and ends in the colon. The best way to manage any illness is to attend to colon health. Proper elimination, digestion, and absorption of nutrients are a major buffer against organ degeneration, apart from psychosomatic stress. Cleansing of the large intestine with liquids is an *enema*. It is a procedure that has been in practice for over 4,000 years. It is a ritual in the treatment of degenerative diseases. It is especially important today because of the consumption of processed foods, foods grown with chemicals, and food devoid of fiber. An enema involves administration of liquid at low pressure into the rectum trough the anus to induce bowel movement. It washes and cleanses the colon, re-populates the colon with pro-biotic organisms, and is used to treat digestive disease, to re-hydrate the body through the colon, and to remove accumulated fecal matter. An enema taken with a professional colon therapist is referred to as a colonic, and an enema taken on a colema board is known as a *colema*. I recommend Dr. Bernard Jensen's guide to better bowel care as a guide on how to do a colema with a colema board. A colon hydrotherapy session should last an average of about 30 – 45 minutes.

Why is Colon Hydrotherapy Significant?

Colon hydrotherapy is a safe and easy way to clean the colon of old accumulated wastes.
Hardened fecal matter and mucus lining the walls of the intestine reduces the ability of nutrients from the intestine to go to the liver. This impairment leads to craving for more food and craving for more flavors. Colon hydrotherapy breaks this vicious cycle by
- removing harmful toxins from the gut;
- stimulating the immune system;
- allowing absorption and assimilation of nutrients;
- preventing auto-intoxication
- enhancing peristalsis;
- eliminating colonization of harmful bacteria;
- normalizing bowel movements; and
- Takes stress off of the liver.

Doing Colonic with a Therapist

This basically involves the passage of purified warm water into all segments of the colon through the rectum by a colon hydro-therapist while the patient lies on their back down or side. It is basically safe and effective in relieving wastes from the colon. It normally lasts between 30 – 45 minutes after an initial 10 – 15 minute session. Bi-weekly sessions are recommended to effectively address most long-standing health concerns and to eliminate fecal matter that has accumulated since childhood. Each session cost between 50 and 75 dollars. During colonic irrigation, the therapist massages the stomach area to facilitate the relaxation of the abdominal muscles and make sure all parts of the colon are evenly irrigated. During the session, the inflow and outflow of low-pressure water in the colon is controlled by the therapist. As the water leaves the colon, the wastes can be viewed by both the client and the therapist.

Colon hydrotherapy goes deeper into the colon than enemas. Enemas primarily address the rectal area, but if price is a concern it is also advisable. Enema kits are available in most health foods stores and pharmaceutical stores. Studies indicate that one colon hydrotherapy session is equivalent to having about 25 enemas.

A home enema kit from a drug store of health food store should include disposable non-latex rubber gloves, an enema tube, bag, nozzle or tip, and clamps or a stop cock. You may use any of the following liquids for an enema:

- Filtered or distilled water (Distilled water help pull toxins out of the body. Since it is devoid of nutrients, distilled water pulls nutrients and toxins toward the colon to facilitate detoxification. Please don't use tap water.)
- pro-biotics to replenish the colon with friendly bacteria
- extra virgin organic olive oil
- herbal teas

Procedure for Doing a Home Enema
- Allocate a private area in a spacious bathroom with a well-draped floor or bed. Connect the enema bag with the enema tube and the enema tube with the enema nozzle and stopcock.
- Fill the enema bag with about two quarts of filtered mildly warm fluids.

- Hang the enema bag about 4 feet (1 – 1.5 meters) above the rectum to allow gravity to push the liquid slowly down. If the bag is held too high, colon spasms can occur.
- Lubricate the enema rectal tip with water-soluble KY jelly or Vaseline.
- Lay on your back on the floor.
- Inset the lubricated enema rectal tip into the rectum, release the clamp or stopcock and let the liquid flow gently into the large intestine (colon). If possible, retain the enema for 3 – 10 minutes. If pain occurs, clamp off the liquid flow and allow the sensation to end before resuming. A slow fill allows more warm liquid to fill the entire colon.
- Gently massage the abdomen in a counterclockwise direction to moves the liquid farther into the colon. If there is a need to evacuate, release into the toilet.
- After emptying your bowel you can repeat the process until you empty the enema bag.

COFFEE RETENTION ENEMA

Autopsies have shown that the bowel can become lined with accumulated material just like an old sewer pipe, in some cases to the point where the opening is no larger in diameter than a pencil.

When used as a retention enema—an enema that is held in the body for a specified period of time—a coffee enema does not go through the digestive system, and does not affect the body as a coffee beverage does. Instead, the coffee solution stimulates both the liver and the gallbladder to release toxins, which are then flushed from the body. A coffee-retention enema is quite helpful during a serious illness, after hospitalization, and after exposure to toxic chemicals. This enema can also be used during fasts to relieve the headaches sometimes caused by a fast-induced release of toxins. Caffeine contains theophylline and theobromine that combine to stimulate the relaxation of smooth muscles causing dilatation of blood vessels and bile ducts. The caffeine is absorbed more quickly and in higher concentration through the enterohepatic circulation than it is in when coffee is taken through the mouth. This allows the liver and the gallbladder to almost immediately dump all the bile and toxins that they were holding. This creates a deficit in the toxic load of the liver relative to the whole body, so that toxins from other areas of the body are attracted to the liver to fill the vacuum created. The liver, being relived of its toxic load, can then effectively excrete the toxins.

The effects of having a coffee enema are not the same as drinking coffee. The enzymes in coffee, known as palmitates, help the liver carry away the toxins in bile acid. This enzyme gets the liver to produce an enzyme that cleans the blood. Tests show that during a coffee enema, the liver will produce up to 700 percent more of this enzyme than it normally would. The veins of the anus are very close to the surface of the tissue, so the coffee is absorbed into the hemorrhoidal vein, then taken up to the liver by the portal vein. With the bile ducts dilated, bile carries toxins away to the gastro-intestinal tract. Simultaneously, peristaltic activity is encouraged because of the flooding of the lower colon. Thus, when the colon is evacuated, the toxins and bile are carried out of the body. A squealing sound is often heard after about 30 minutes, announcing the release of toxins from the liver, gall bladder, and bile duct after the coffee enema is done. Individuals who are allergic to caffeine might want to use a lemon juice enema instead.

Organic herbal retention enemas involve a combination of any given herb or juices administered with professional approval. The advantages of herbal-retention enemas are numerous. The herbs do not have to pass through harsh acidic conditions in the stomach which degrade their nutritional contents. Like rectal suppositories that are used to achieve a therapeutic effect, herbal-retention enemas are absorbed directly into systemic circulation through the rectum. Some people do not like the flavor of herbal infusions and may thus try them as enemas. The mucous membrane of the bowels can absorb the original active substances from a liquid injected as an enema much faster and better than taking them orally.

When doing a coffee enema, use three or four tablespoons of ground drip organic coffee to one quart of water. Let the entire mixture boil for three minutes and then simmer 20 minutes more. Strain and let the water cool to body temperature. Then pour the coffee liquid into the enema bag. Never utilize flavored coffee, sweetened coffee, or coffee with milk (*cafe au lait*) for this purpose. Excess use of coffee enemas over a 6-month period may deplete the body's stores of iron and other minerals, vitamins, and can cause anemia. Do not use coffee enemas for more than four months at a time.

To make enemas the most effective, the patient should lie on their right side with both legs drawn up close to the abdomen. Try to hold the enema in for 5 – 20 minutes. Some people use a plastic sheet on the floor "just in case" or put a diaper pad where you lay. You might try lying on a beach towel on the bathroom floor while massaging the abdomen. Stay close to a toilet, though, because the coffee does cause peristaltic contractions and the results are marvelously effective. After an enema session, it is important to clean the rectal tip with bleach and soap and water to avoid infections. To avoid infection, enema kits should not be shared with other people.

How do I know if my colon is clean?
The color of the water coming out will tell you if your colon is clean. You have to be patient with yourself. The French fries you ate 20 years ago might still be in there. Most people have layers of muciod plaques caked to the walls of the colon. It will take lots of lubrications for liquids to seep into them, soften them, and peel them off the walls of the colon. It may take weeks of repeated enemas to get them out.

Doctor's health Advisory: Herbal enemas should be administered with professional approval. Enemas should be done with great care and lubrication so as not to rupture the rectum. Also, frequent colonic irrigation often leads to electrolyte leaching that could disturb the body's electrolyte balance. This can be avoided with adequate use pro-biotic organisms or adequate consumption of organic foods rich in pro-biotics, sodium, potassium, and magnesium which will help re-establishes electrolyte balance.

+ *Flashback*
Westernization of traditional life has made my health too sedentary for my metabolism. As previously noted, the ancients liken the human body to an irrigation system that is traversed by three great rivers. Like the Amazon River that self-cleanses itself by its flow, so also does the human body. The red river or the cardiovascular carries the red blood cells. It is propagated into motion as the heart pumps and as we engage in physical activity. The white river is the lymphatic system that carries the white blood cells that are also propagated by physical movement. The alimentary canal functions under the influences of gravity, and requires wholesome food for effective bowel movements. Stagnation in any or all of these systems is thought to be the etiology of organ degeneration

Like borrowing new money to pay old debt, I used stronger and newer anti-virals and chemotherapy drugs that made me indebted to newer symptoms. My orthodox approach to health emphasized the pathology over my physiology. I needed a paradigm shift to a road less traveled. Health and happiness that eluded me were stored but unreleased within me. Like the proverbial prodigal son who veered from his inheritance through ignorance, my unhappy state was due to violation of natural laws of health. Like Francis Bacon rightfully said, "for nature to be commanded, it has to be obeyed." In search of the American dream, I got to the point where my material wants exceeded my needs. I was estranged from the self that never lived in me. I realized that forgiveness is up to me and not by those who have transgressed against me. I needed light in my tunnel as liver disease and cancer had made me jaundiced like mustard. I was passing through the dark nights, with the winds against my soul. I was no longer at ease until I veered from medical orthodoxy to the path that led to a trail of alternatives. There I found health and the tree of life that was always planted in me.

Moving Bile with the Liver and Gall Bladder Flush

"The liver – gall bladder cleanse is an age-old procedure that helps the liver empty its contents into the colon for excretion. It is a way to dump old bile, bile soaps, hardened bile, and gallstones into the colon. This gives the liver system a new energy for a fresh start." JackTipps

The gallbladder is a sack in the liver. Its functions are intricately related to that of the liver. It is the reservoir of the bile salts that emulsify fats and metabolize fat soluble vitamins. Bile thus helps as a means to effectively eliminate toxins from the body. Similarly, bile helps to synthesis fat soluble vitamins (Vitamins A, D, E, and K) in the intestine and improves their absorption. Each day, about one quart of bile is manufactured by the liver, and it serves as a carrier of toxic substances that are dumped into the intestine. These toxic substances are absorbed by fiber and excreted. Low-fiber diets lead to inadequate binding and re-absorption of toxins. This becomes problematic when intestinal bacteria modify these toxins to more virulent forms. A toxic liver will cause an inflamed gall bladder; the bile salts crystallize and form gallstones. In this situation, fat metabolism is impaired and toxicity is heightened. This necessitates the need for the liver – gall bladder cleanse. Getting rid of the gallstones and keeping the gall bladder healthy are necessary for optimal liver health and preferable to surgical removal of the gall bladder.

Cholestasis, one of the indications for a need for a liver – gall bladder cleanse, is a liver disease caused by disruption of the flow of bile through the bile duct in any part of the bilary system. This is due to the presence of gallstones, drug side effects, steroids, tumors, alcohol use, or other inflammation-causing agents. Cholestasis causes abnormalities in liver function and affects the liver enzymes and functioning. The level of serum bile acids are used to diagnose cholestasis. It is corrected with surgery to facilitate flow. It is also resolved if the underlying inflammations and drug use are addressed.

Preparing for a Flush
To prepare for a gall bladder – liver cleanse, one needs to eliminate vegetable and hydrogenated oils, cheese, white sugar, white bread, white rice, processed foods, alcohol, nicotine, fried foods, processed foods, red meat, pasteurized milk and milk products, eggs, greasy foods, margarine, caffeine, sodas, pastas, cereals, and coffee from their diets for about one week preceding the flush, and eat more fruits and vegetables during that time. Also, drink about one quart of apple juice and/or herbal teas daily throughout the week preceding the flush to help soften the gall stones and facilitate their passage from the gall bladder. Moving towards a diet centered on steamed vegetables will start the cleansing before the actual flush, too.

On the day of the flush, drink about 6-8 glasses of liquids, including juices, soups, water, and tea. Additionally, you need to take about 6 glasses of lemon, apple juice, lime, or grapefruit juice to help dissolve the gall stones. These liquids help dilate the gall bladder and bile ducts so the stones and materials can spill easily into the digestive tract where they are eliminated. I recommend avoiding solid food throughout the day of the flush.

Before going to bed, drink 6-8 ounces of organic extra virgin organic olive oil, which constricts the gall bladder, helping it to eliminate the gallstones, and half a cup of organic lemon, apple, or grapefruit juice, which help dissolve the gallstones. Finally, I recommend taking two teaspoons of Epsom salts dissolved in about 5 tablespoons of water. Crisscrossing the architecture of the liver is a densely packed web of passageways called the bile ducts which drain into the gall bladder. The Epsom salts will help dilate the gall bladder bile ducts so the stones and contents can move out more easily. The presence of large amounts of olive oil in the intestines tricks the liver into stimulating emulsification, by which the gall bladder will secrete bile and accumulated toxins into the digestive tract. Take a warm bath, which will also help dilate the bile ducts, and sleep on the right side to help facilitate drainage of bile.

The following day, drink regular fruit and vegetable juices or the super food formulas, and watch for the presence of gallstone when you use the bathroom. What you see might surprise you.

Doctors Health Advisory: I recommend doing the liver – gall bladder cleansing biennially. It is advisable not to use the bile-moving herbs during the liver – gallbladders cleanse to avoid multiplication of effects. The bile-moving herbs can be taken after the cleanse. Individuals diagnosed with gallstones should not immediately do the gall bladder flush because the olive oil constricts the gall bladder to eliminate the gallstone. It is advised to dissolve the gallstone first with lemon, lime, and/or apple juice for a few months before doing the flush. Similarly, those who have had their gall bladders removed can still do the flush to relieve the load on the liver since they still have their bile ducts for toxins to flow through.

Diabetics may not use apple juice because of the high sugar content and those who are hypertensive may not use the grape fruit juice.

It is advisable to do colonic irrigation or an enema immediately following the flush. If the bowel is toxic when the liver and gall bladder is being detoxified, the body will suffer from toxic overload which can cause nausea, vomiting, and headaches as the body tries to get rid of the liver toxins. When the bowel is clean, toxins will move freely through to the rectum.

The difference between the bile-moving herbs and the gall bladder flush is that the bile moving herbs have dual actions: They move bile and cleanse the blood of impurities simultaneously. They are referred to as systemic blood cleansers. A coffee enema is also very useful when we want to flush bile from the liver and gallbladder

⊠ *Flashback*
Though my liver enzymes were within normal limits, I was not whole. I realized that being well is totally different from being whole. According to C.J Jung, the

211

attainment of wholeness requires one to stake ones whole being. Nothing less will do, there can be no easier conditions, no substitutes, no compromises. The word "health" is derived from the old Teutonic word meaning "salvation." This entails the body, the mind, and the spirit as a whole. Being whole entails being healed from within. I had unresolved resentments and unforgiving attitudes that made wholeness elude me. Like Booker T. Washington, I need not allow any man to reduce my mind to the level of hatred any more. I realized that we are not angered by adversities but by adversities perceived as injuries. I drew a lot of inspiration from Johann Wolfgang Goethe who indicated in one of his writings that "until one is committed, there is hesitancy, the chance to draw back, always ineffectiveness…The moment one definitely commits ones self, then providence moves too. All sorts of things occur to help one that would never otherwise have occurred." I had to stop viewing life from other people's rationalizations. I realized that while old established mindsets cannot be erased, they can be replaced with positive reinforcements, imaginations, and affirmations. I took a clue from the motto of the United Negro College Fund that says "a mind is a terrible thing to waste." My thoughts formed things I did not like, and my moods took me to mental places that hindered my healing. I realized that energy is a neutral force that is directed to forms by our thoughts, and my negative thought patterns were negating my desire to be whole. The only things in our lives over which we have control are our thoughts and our actions caused by them. I realized that the body only manifests what we believe and what the mind thinks the body thinks and that which the body thinks it actualizes. Preparing my mind to a condition that defies illness becomes my pre-occupation. The more I reached in and let go of these emotions, the more my physical health rebounded to heights I had never imagined. I had gotten to the point that I had to love and die or love and heal, and I choose the latter. Negativity was draining the healing currents that flowed endlessly through my thoughts. As I learned to avoid being sapped by my attachments to negative emotions or to other peoples negative energies, false symbols, or power (e.g. money and external authority), my sense of inner peace improved. The more I sought divine presence in my life, the more His essence became my purpose. I developed a purpose-driven life. My values changed. I had accepted my self completely and hepatitis doesn't scare me any more. Herbs made me well but love made me whole.

Chapter 11

Lifestyles for a Healthy Liver

In 1874, Dr. Andrew Still in Missouri proposed that illness was caused by stagnation of vital bodily functions. He believed that when we stimulate the lymphatic and cardiovascular systems and eliminate sluggishness, most illness will be eradicated. Just like stagnant water will cause destructive sedimentation and corrosion to its container, stagnation and a sedentary lifestyle will cause organ degeneration. Proponent of orthodox medicine pounced on him and his osteopathic colleagues and put them in jail for their convictions. How wrong were they? Today doctors of osteopathic medicines have become household names in the American medicine.

Significance of the Lymphatic and Respiratory systems

One of the major causes of chronic degenerative diseases is internal pollution. When organs and tissues do not get adequate supplies of oxygen, they cannot utilize nutrients, and tissue death ensues. Similarly, their inability to rid themselves of cellular wastes and debris compound the problem of cellular degeneration. The consequences of these stagnations are what lead to reduced immunity to diseases. In the presence of oxygen, cellular wastes and toxins are broken down and passed out through the blood and the kidneys.

A general understanding of the lymphatic system will buttress the need for lymphatic massage, deep breathing, and physical exercise for detoxification. It plays a crucial role in the body's ability to ward off illnesses and recover from diseases. The lymphatic system is twice the size of the circulatory system. Like the cardiovascular system, movement is key to its optimal functioning, and sluggishness leads to its failure. Like a house with two plumbing systems, the lymphatic system runs parallel to the vascular system. While the cardiovascular system supplies blood and nutrients to the tissues, the lymphatic system runs side by side to the vascular system to collect the leftover intracellular wastes for purification, filtration, and recycling. Nature puts this system in place to offset the danger of tissue wastes hanging around the body. It is often referred to as the body's sewage disposal system.

When the lymphatic system becomes stagnant with wastes, debris, cellular wastes, dietary fats, and toxins, the usually-clear lymphatic fluid becomes thick with mucus. The failure of the lymphatic system leads to a wide variety of issues, from head aches to cancer. This is like what happens when the garbage disposal workers go on strike—a mess ensues! The blood vessels carry oxygen-rich blood from the heart to the arteries and the capillaries from which they diffuse into the tissues and organs, which extract nutrients and oxygen from the capillaries for their well being. In exchange, they excrete their by-products and toxins to the capillaries.

While the circulatory system uses blood to supply oxygen and nutrients to all body organs, the lymphatic system uses the lymph fluid to access body tissues. If the activity of the lymphatic system is stopped, death occurs in a matter of hours. It filters toxins as fluids move through it, and it manufactures antibodies to neutralize antigens. It receives excess fluids and proteins that the capillary and vascular system leave behind which would cause swelling in the tissues. The lymphatic system is twice the size of the vascular system. The vascular system has the heart as its central pump but the lymphatic system needs breathing, physical exercise, movement of the extremities, and muscular action to move substances through the body to empty its contents.

The lymph nodes are located in places like the arms, legs, torso, and neck where there is frequent movement. They appear like pearls knotted on a string. Like small streams trickling into a large river, the lymphatic fluids converge to the lymph nodes as collection points. While the purification process goes on, the lymphatic fluids travel up the torso, through the thoracic duct along the left side of the esophagus. There, it merges with the lymphatic system from the left trunk and the arm and eventually returns its purified contents to the blood stream at its junction with the left subclavican vein above the heart under the collar bone. Lesser and smaller volumes of the filtered lymphatic fluids travel from the nodes along the right side of the head, neck, and arm are returned back to the blood stream via the right lymphatic duct on the right side of the collar bone.

If there are blockages in the lymph nodes, there is a back up that results in accumulation of toxins. This is often referred to as lymph edema. This leads to stagnation in the interstitial tissue space and impairment of lymph flow through the lymph vessels. Circulation and supply of nutrients to the organs and tissues are hampered from lymphatic stagnation. The accumulation of toxins from lymphatic stagnation is implicated in a wide variety of chronic degenerative diseases.

An important function of the lymph tissue is manufacture and storage of infection-fighting white blood cells. Aside from the lymph nodes, other principal lymph organs are the bone marrow that manufactures the B lymphocytes, the tonsils, the spleen, and the thymus that manufactures the T lymphocytes. Lymphoma is a cancer related to the lymphocytes. The largest aggregation of lymph tissues in the body surrounds the digestive tract. They are called gut-associated lymph tissue (GALT). It is through the digestive system that the majority of pathogens that afflict humanity enter systemic circulation. While the beneficial bacteria in the gut, enzymes, and acids in the system try to neutralize these pathogens, many sail through to the waiting arms of GALT. The GALT is on its own in coordinating immune responses from the gut. This characteristic has earned it the name "the second brain." Problems often arise when the blood is dumping toxins from the gut into the lymphatic system via the liver. The lymphatic system becomes overworked and its filtration and neutralizing ability is hampered. A toxic bowel leaks toxins into smaller veins that gradually join together until they form one larger vein called the portal vein which goes to the liver directly. The lymphatic fluids, now filled with toxins, are absorbed into the lymphatic system and drained into the blood via the thoracic duct.

The Significance of Deep Breathing
Naturally, physical inactivity makes the lymphatic fluids move slowly and compounds stagnation. During breathing, our body exchange about 12,000 quarts of air daily. Deep breathing activates the lymphatic system. It depends on breathing and skeletal muscle contraction to move its fluids through the body. Breathing, as a form of detoxification, drives the lymphatic drainage. When we take deep breaths and exhale deeply, we are massaging the thoracic duct upward into the neck, making it easy for

lymphatic fluids to flow into the venous blood. Yawning is the natural urge of the body to do deep breathing, because carbon dioxide build up and the brain stimulate people to take a deep breath to get rid of carbon dioxide. The breathing process makes the lymphatic system drain its contents into the veins where they become part of the blood plasma. From there, the lymph contents are returned to the liver and the kidney for filtration. The tissues extract nutrients from the oxygenated blood and excrete toxins back to the capillaries which are removed by the lymphatic system.

The lymphatic system is activated by deep breathing. It prevents life-threatening back ups of toxins. Deep breathing rids the body of these toxic by-products of cellular metabolism during detoxification. Lack of oxygen leads to tissue hypoxia, reduced ability of the body to throw off toxins, and loss of vitality. During breathing, the cells exhale carbonic acid, which turns to carbon dioxide. This is passed out through the lungs, thereby reducing the acid load of the body and moving the body towards a more healthy alkaline state (Colbin, 1998). Oxygen derived from breathing is a universal cleanser. High levels of oxygen helps in the break down of cellular wastes. Most viruses, bacteria, and all cancerous cells utilize anaerobic metabolism; they thrive best in environments where oxygen is deficient. When there is an increase in the oxygen supply to tissues, microbes cannot multiply and cancerous cells cannot thrive. They are destroyed outright. Oxygenated blood from the lungs is pivotal to the metabolic and catabolic activities of the liver. Oxygen makes up 90 percent of the weight of water. Vitamin C needs oxygen for the breakdown of collagen (Pitchford, 2002). Oxygen is also delivered to the tissues via raw fruits and vegetable juices.

A Simple Deep-Breathing Exercise
The average person breaths about 23,000 times daily to nourish the over 100 trillion cells in the body. Every passing minute, 300 million cells die and new ones are produced. Taking time off to do deep breathing can make a big difference in the quality of new cells being produced when making a transition from sickness to health. We want to ensure that the newer cells do not follow the pattern of the older diseased cells. During breathing, the hemoglobin is able to carry oxygen rich cells to deeper areas for oxidation.

Because indoor air is about 70 times more toxic than outdoor air in major cities, deep breathing is preferable outdoors if possible. The exercise should

be about five minutes in a comfortable sitting position about four times daily in the following pattern:
- Inhale for a count of 4 or about 5 seconds.
- Hold for a count of 10 or about 15 seconds.
- Exhale for a count of 5 or about 6 seconds.

During inhalation, the diaphragm is filled with air while the rib cage moves up and the stomach moves outward. During exhalation, the diaphragm move up and the stomach moves inward. These movements facilitate the movement of lymphatic fluid to the drainage channels. Inhaling air with the stomach moving in or exhaling air with the stomach moving out is counterproductive.

Why Lymphatic Massage?

Lymphatic massage therapy helps stimulate the lymphatic system and facilitates lymphatic elimination during detoxification. It also reduces physical and mental tension. Lymphatic massage serves to drain excess fluids that flow into the lymphatic system's filtering stations and to flush waste matter, preventing or reducing its escape into the blood stream. It also allows sticky, toxic mucus from the tissues to be dumped into the colon for elimination, since the colon is the principle organ through which mucus from the lymphatic system is eliminated. When the body is producing toxins at a rate greater than it can process them, the body protects us by suspending these toxins in fat and interstitial spaces. This result in an excess build up of lymph fluids in the lymphatic system.

Saunas: The Sweat Therapy

Fog, high rise buildings, cell phone towers, and greenhouse gases have caused environmental pollution by blocking the healing essence of infrared rays from reaching mankind. Infrared rays are one of the beneficial invisible rays that comes from sunlight. When it penetrates the skin, it transforms light energy into heat energy. It heats the body without increasing the temperature. This results in a much lower power bill when compared to traditional steam saunas. Infrared saunas are a form of sweat therapy that help eliminate large amounts of toxins and uric acid from the blood, which ultimately reduces the livers work load. Infrared saunas detoxify the body at the cellular level rather than just detoxifying the sweat glands. It penetrates about 3 inches deep in the skin. The penetration of such healing rays into the tissues subsequently facilitates circulation of blood and lymphatic flow. This leads naturally to the release of toxins from their stores through the fat cells, the sweat glands, the skin, the liver, and the kidney. It enhances the function of the largest organ of detoxification in the body, the skin, by bypassing the kidney, the liver, and the lungs. High temperatures dilate the blood vessels, and the circulation in the skin increases as it takes deeply buried toxins to the skin's surface. Saunas help the body to perspire and help move toxins from inside to outside. Heat releases toxins from the cells and tissues into the lymphatic system. Since sweat is manufactured from lymphatic fluid, toxins from the lymph are released when sweating occurs.

There are two types of saunas: infrared (convection) and conventional saunas. Infrared saunas are superior to conventional saunas. They use only about 20 percent of the infrared energy to heat the air, and the remaining 80 percent is converted to heat within the body. The net result is more and quicker perspiration and more penetration at lower temperatures of about 110 – 130°F. It also produces more sweat volume. It usually lasts for 30 – 45 minutes per session (Watson, 2006). Conventional saunas use external sources of heat to raise the temperature to 180 – 235°F. Burning wood or an electrical source is used to provide the energy that elicits the perspiration, which ultimately helps increase the cardiac load as in aerobic exercise. Thirty minutes in an infrared sauna will burn calories equivalent to a whole day of aerobic exercise. However, saunas do not take the place of physical exercise.

Doctors Health Advisory: Saunas do not take the place of sunlight. We still need sunlight to supply us with UV and convert vitamins to usable forms in the body. Infrared saunas are contraindicated in pregnant women.

Will Exposure to Sunlight Cause Me to get Skin Cancer?
The correlation between sunlight and skin cancer is contentious. We definitely need sunlight to shrink cancer cells and convert vitamin D to usable forms. Moderation is the key if you produce melanin more rapidly than others. About 30 minutes under the sun daily will do more good than anything else to your health. Sun-block lotions give the skin protection from melanin-producing UV radiation but not from other frequencies of the Sun's radiation that may be equally dangerous to individuals who are predisposed to skin cancer. While it is generally believed that over exposure to sunlight causes skin cancer, studies indicate that the major culprit is

malnutrition. Though the sun may cause recurrent skin inflammation that leads to cancer in some individuals, malnutrition hampers the body's ability to heal and repair the skin from inflammations. When our dietary patterns are right, we should have anti-inflammatory and anti-oxidant protection against all cancers (Malkmus and Shockey, 2006).

Dry skin brushing cleans the skin of old and dead cells and debris so that toxins can move out without hindrances. The skin is the largest eliminative organ. It works with the colon, the kidney, and the lungs to rid the body of by products of metabolic wastes and toxins. Since we make a new top layer of skin every 24 hours, it is necessary to consciously brush away the old top layer to let the new top layer come to the surface (Jensen, 1999). It is crucial in ridding the body of toxins. Studies indicate that the skin helps take out more than two pound of wastes daily from the human body in the form of perspiration. This necessitates the need to assist the skin in its eliminative actions. Dry skin brushing is one of the means to assist the skin to eliminate toxins. By brushing the skin, we stimulate the sweat glands, facilitate the circulatory system that supplies the tissues and organ systems, open up the pores on the skin, and make it easy for the skin to breathe and eliminate toxins. The blood regularly brings wastes to the skin and skin brushing helps to open the pores and facilitate the elimination of toxins. The whitish, scaly powder-like substance that comes off the skin during brushing is crystals of uric acid and other toxic wastes brought to the surface through perspiration (Jensen, 1999).

Doctor's health advisory: I recommend using a natural-brittle brush from a health food store. It should be kept dry all the time and used in the morning before taking a shower. Brush for 5 – 10 minutes all over the body including hard-to-reach places.

What are the Benefits of Physical Exercise for Liver Patients?

- Have you ever taken time out to look at the clarity of the water in a flowing stream and a stagnant lake? The stagnant lake is always murky with impurities and sedimentations, while a flowing stream looks like spring water. In most rural communities, the water department uses water from springs for public consumption with little or no treatment, while in cities where waters from lakes are being used they are treated with chemicals that threaten the survival of mankind. If

219

you want to flow like a river instead of stagnate like a lake you have to exercise. To aid detoxification, physical exercise enhances lymphatic flow and drainage. It turns stagnation into locomotion. By enhancing lymphatic system flow, we take toxic wastes from the tissues to the veins. From there, they are sent to the liver and kidney for elimination. Also, by enhancing lymphatic flow we enhance the activities of the immune system associated with the lymphatic system (T lymphocytes). These are very critical to liver patients.

- By bypassing the kidney and other eliminative channels, physical exercise initiates sweating and release of toxins and uric acid through the skin.
- During physical exercise, the level of interleukin-6, an inflammatory messenger and one of the key drivers in chronic inflammatory diseases throughout the body, is suppressed (Chilton, 2006).
- Physical exercise, glucose utilization shifts to the muscles and prevents the onset and metastasis of cancer. Cancer cells need glucose to survive.
- Physical exercise boosts cellular oxygenation to tissues which is detrimental to cancer and organ degeneration. Oxygenation is fatal to cancer cells, too.
- Physical exercise enhances the cardiovascular system.
- Exercise help cut down on body fat.
- Physical exercise helps relieve mental stress and increase brain activities, since it helps to send more oxygen rich cells to the brain.

Doctor's health advisory:
The best form of exercise is making something you enjoy a hobby. Drink more water during physical exercise. For every one hour of exercise, it is recommended that you take an extra quart of water. Individuals with liver disease should do light aerobic exercise and weight-bearing exercises about three times a week. Individuals are advised to join a health or physical fitness club to get professional assistance. We advise that before embarking on any type of physical exercise, you should consult with your physician. It is counterproductive to engage in strenuous physical exercise because it leads to reduction of the non-exercise caloric expenditures, and increases desire to eat more (Chilton, 2006).

How much water do I drink?

- The urine output of an average individual is about 1.6 liters daily. We loose additional water during physical activities like breathing, bowel movements, and sweating. Food supplies about 25 percent of our water intake. We need to take in water to counter these losses.
- Water is needed during detoxification to dilute toxins and facilitate their elimination from the body. Dehydration is one of the major causes of diseases. While an average person needs between 6 – 8 glasses (2.2 liter or 74 ounces) of purified water daily to stay healthy, the actual amount of water required depends on the weight and activity level of the individual.
- During detoxification, distilled water is preferable because, being devoid of nutrients; it exhibits solvent effects by pulling toxins from the cells and tissues.
- To find your recommended water intake, divide your weight in pounds by two. The resulting number is the number of water, in ounces, required for a day. For example, a person who weighs 160 pounds will require 80 ounces of water daily. If you use the metric system, divide your weight in kilograms by 30. For example, a 90 kg individual will need 3 liters of water daily. The United States National Research Council recommends 1 mL of water for every calorie you eat. If a person eats 1,000 calories, they should drink 1,000 mL or one liter of water. Water is essential to every major bodily function. This includes circulation of nutrients to all the cells, lubrication of all bodily organs, elimination of toxins, metabolism of fats, and maintenance. During detoxification, water helps dilute and carry end products like nitrogenous waste and urea from liver to the kidney. This reduces the work load of distressed or cirrhotic livers. Just like plants which wither without water, similarly the human cells need to be bathed with water to grow. Without adequate consumption of water during detoxification, toxins are reabsorbed into the tissues.
- Warm water on the body enhances the movement of blood towards the surface of the skin, where it discharges impurities through the relaxed and open pores which are washed off by constant flow of water.

Doctor's Health Advisory: Individuals with high blood pressure decompensated liver cirrhosis, kidney problems, or who have had kidney transplants need to consult with their health care provider before raising their water intake.

What is water intoxication?

A condition known as hyponatremia is a potentially dangerous condition associated with drinking too much water beyond the individual's capacity. The kidney cannot remove the water fast enough so the salt in the blood becomes more dilute. Normally, the amount of water in the body is a tightly-controlled homeostatic ally to the amount of salt in the body. Excessive consumption of water reduces the salt concentration in the blood more than in the cells, and water moves in from the diluted blood to the cells, causing the cells to swell. Swelling in the brain cells causes headaches and disrupts the control of vital functions like breathing. This water intoxication occurs if we go on binge drinking or drinking several liters of water over a very short period of time.

How safe is your tap water?

"Cities across the United States, such as Philadelphia, Boston, and New York City, were manipulating the results of tests used to detect lead in water, violating Federal law and putting millions of Americans at risk by giving them a false sense of security." October 5th*, 2004 issue of the Washington Post.*

The public water supply in the United States is not safe for human consumption. Consequently, most people rely on different filtration systems to get clean drinking water. Livestock consume about half of the U.S. water supply (Kunjufu, 2000). About 6.8 billion gallons of water are flushed down U.S. toilets daily (Graves, 2006). Since most water is consumed by livestock, sewage water contaminated with bacteria, human excrement, and chemicals are recycled to tap water in large American cities. Chemical are added to city water to keep the pipes from rusting. These chemicals are detrimental to the health of humans. Most cities add chlorine to disinfect the water and sodium fluoride for tooth-decay prevention. Chlorine is metabolized to chloroform in the body. Fluoric acid is the chemical added to city water supplies (Pitchford, 2002). Fluorine is a vitamin and enzyme inhibitor (Anderson and Jensen1990). It is classified as a drug, a poison, and an industrial waste product of the aluminum and fertilizer industries, controlled at one time by the Mellon family. It pollutes the air, damages wild life and livestock, and endangers humanity.

These substances were initially disposed of by being sold as rat poison and insecticide. Later, there weren't enough insects and rats to poison. Also, fluoride is not biodegradable and its excessive use as an insecticide and rodenticide could create health hazards for humanity. Its disposal became a problem for the industrial-agricultural complex. The problem was solved by dumping this waste into public drinking water, and the public was told it reduced tooth decay. The American dental association and the U.S.Public Health Service authorized this bureaucratic policy to counter public welfare. The CDC estimates that 30,000 – 50,000 people die each year in the U.S. where 1 part per million of fluoride is added to public drinking water. There may be no safe level for fluoride to exert its deleterious effects on the human body. Evidence shows that fluoride causes dental fluorosis, tooth decay, and increased tooth loss. Fluoride tricks, damages, and disarms the immune system. It alters the shapes of proteins, the building blocks of the immune system. When the shapes of proteins are altered, the body sees them as foreign bodies and attacks them. This is one of the etiologies of autoimmune diseases, inflammatory diseases, and allergies. Fluorides decrease the ability of white blood cells to migrate to areas of infection. Fluoride inhibits enzymatic reactions in the body by binding to enzyme co-factors. It disrupts the hydrogen bonds that help proteins maintain their normal shapes, thereby disrupting the enzymatic activities of proteins whose ability to trigger a reaction is highly dependent on a shape stabilized by hydrogen bonds. In addition, the disruption of the hydrogen bonding of the DNA molecule by fluoride causes tremendous damage to the human genome. A family-size fluoridated tooth paste, weighing about 7 ounces contain 100 parts per million fluoride can kill a small child weighing up to 20 pounds (Yiamouyiannis, 1986).

Chlorine combines with other organic substance that may be in the water to form chloroform, a poisonous substance that does not evaporate. Chlorine interferes with the metabolism of vitamin E in the body (Pitchford, 2002). It is used as an antiseptic in public tap water and all swimming pools. Aluminum, which causes a wide variety of human afflictions, is added to public water to make it sparkle (Baroody, 2002). The use of aluminum cookware is unsafe, as it contributes heavy metals to tissues and puts tremendous stress on the immune system.

Doctors Health advisory: Drink more fluids during the day because drinking more fluids after 8 pm might result in waking up in the night to urinate. This might disrupt a refreshing sleep. It is best to avoid drinking at least two hours before bedtime.

To improve the quality of water you drink, the following recommendations might be helpful:

- Avoid drinking distilled water regularly, since it is devoid of nutrients and draws on the body's reserves of nutrients and deplete the body's needed minerals.
- Check bottled water carefully because most of it is not spring water but purified tap water.
- If possible install a reverse-osmosis filtration system in your house. This is about the best home system at this time. Other systems that use charcoal, ceramic, or high quality filters are also acceptable. The goal is to reduce the contamination from heavy metals, fluorine, chlorine, microorganisms, and other contaminants.
- Drink warm or room-temperature water. Digestion functions best when we drink warm water. It is best to drink water about 30 minutes before or after food. Drinking water while eating dilutes the digestive juices and reduces the efficacy. Traditional Chinese medicine teaches that cold water disrupts the flow of energy in the body and "shocks" the body.

Is hydrogenated Oil and Vegetable Oil Good for you?

Oil Processing
Several different steps and methods are used in the processing of oils. The quality, flavor, and nutritional content of oils varies greatly according to which processes are used.

Extraction
How oil is extracted affects the nutritional quality of the oil because heat, light, and oxygen can destroy nutrients. Here are the most commonly used extraction methods:

Expeller pressing — a process that uses mechanical pressure rather than chemicals to extract oil from its source. Friction generates temperatures that may be as high as 185°F depending on the hardness of the seed, grain, bean, or nut.

Cold pressing — the term sometimes used for expeller pressing at temperatures below 120°F. A common cold-pressed oil is extra virgin olive oil, which comes from the first pressing of olives. The Spectrum brand now cold presses many of its delicate oils, like flax, pumpkin, and hazelnut.

Vacuum extraction — a recently-developed (SpectraVac) vacuum expeller process that extracts oils in a non-oxygen and light-free atmosphere at temperatures as low as 70°F.

Solvent extraction — oils are extracted chemically with petroleum solvents which destroy the oil's nutritional value. Oil processing involves extraction with solvents like hexane or heptane (gasoline) is passed off to consumers as "unrefined oils." They undergo processes like de-guming, bleaching, and deodorizing to produce the final refined product. Important nutrients like fiber, lecithin, and chlorophyll, and metals like magnesium, iron, and copper are lost when oil is refined. Caustic soda and sodium carbonate are used as a base to help remove free fatty acids from oils. Bleaching with the toxic peroxide process removes beta-carotene from unrefined oils. Deodorization takes place at very high temperatures (Erasmus, 1993).

Hydrogenation

Hydrogenation is the chemical process that transforms a liquid oil into a solid or partially-solid form. Hydrogenation of oils changes essential and unsaturated fatty acids into substances that do not spoil and that last forever. It involves the addition of nickel and aluminum, which are toxic to the body. This final product, sold as shortenings, vegetable oils, margarines, corn oil, canola oils, and cottonseed oil are toxic and foreign to the body. They are referred to as trans-fatty acids. They increase our LDL cholesterol, which interferes with enzyme functions and puts undue strain on the liver. These trans-fatty acids are not compatible with the enzymes and membrane structures of humans. They make platelets sticky, increasing the likelihood of blood clots in small blood vessels, they affect enzyme metabolism, they punch holes in cells membranes, and they impair immune function and facilitate organ degeneration (Erasmus, 1993). The process uses heavy metals, hydrogen gas, and extremely high temperatures. Hydrogenation destroys nutrients and transforms the fat into trans-fatty acids. Consuming trans-fatty acids has been linked to high cholesterol and heart disease.

Margarine and shortening are products that have been hydrogenated. Other sources of hydrogenated or partially-hydrogenated oils are packaged snacks like cookies, crackers, chips, and pastries. Look for brands that use natural vegetable oils for a healthier choice. The FDA now requires the total grams of trans-fatty acids to be listed on food packages.

Coconut Oil: Fat That Heals

Coconut oil is a colorless oil extracted from the flesh of coconut. Despite the benefits of coconut oil, the Food and Drug Administration recommend avoiding coconut because it is high in saturated oil. Why has this highly-beneficial oil been so grossly misunderstood? There are lots of saturated oils on the market; coconut is one of the few that heals, and does not kill. Coconut meat has about 8 g of fiber per cup and as much proteins as green beans and carrots, as well as folic acid, calcium, iron, and vitamin B1, B6, C, and E. Unlike other dietary fats that produce body fats, coconut oil produces energy, and, unlike other vegetables oils, it does not oxidize easily because it is resistant to free radical attack.

Coconut oil is a potent natural antibiotic that is effective against the HCV and HIV viruses. It is a natural antibacterial, antiviral, anti-fungal, and anti-protozoal food.

Its anti-microbial properties are derived from its composition of medium-chain fatty acids (MCFA). They are absent from all other vegetable and animal oil except *perm kernel oil*. They are harmless to humans and deadly to viruses. The coconut oil found in fresh coconuts has almost no anti-microbial properties but, when eaten, our bodies break it into triglycerides, monoglycerides, and free fatty acids, which have anti-microbial properties (Fife, 2003). The most active of these are lauric acid, capric acid, and the monoglycerides monolaurin and monocaprin. Lauric acid is also found in breast milk. It also contains caprylic acid that is thought to be a potent antifungal agent. Lauric acid and monolaurin have the greatest antimicrobial effects.

Most bacteria and viruses are lipid coated. The fatty acids that make up their outer membranes are similar to those of the coconut oil MCFA. This similarity facilitates their attraction to the membranes of lipid-coated viruses and bacteria. MCFA of coconut oil are smaller and can penetrate and disrupt the lipid membranes of viruses. They spill the DNA and other cellular material of the virus open, thereby killing the virus. The host's white blood cells then dispose of the cellular debris. Coconut oil is absorbed directly into the liver from the gut where it deactivates the hepatitis C virus. Coconut oil has exciting fat-burning power because of it's concentration of medium-chain triglycerides which, instead of being stored in fat cells, are used for energy production while stimulating metabolism. (Fife, 2003), (Erasmus, 2003), (Karst and Vanderhaeghe, 2004). Because it is a saturated fat, Americans have been brainwashed to link all saturated fats with heart disease without knowing the difference between fats that kill and those that heal, says Erasmus (2003). Most people do not know that coconut oil has medium-chain fatty acids that are different from the saturated fats found in meats and other dietary products. It was part of a calculated campaign by the food-processing industries to replace tropical unprocessed oils with vegetable hydrogenated oils that are embalmed to have eternal shelf life and stay liquid at all temperatures. While they are processed to last forever, they send humans to early graves. The same food processing industries that discouraged the public from using coconut oil secretly isolated and patented genetically-engineered prototypes of its most potent ingredient, lauric acid, for big profits—a classical case of talking out of both sides of the mouth. (Fife, 2003)

Doctors Health Advisory: I recommend taking one teaspoon of organic cold pressed extra virgin coconut oil about three to four times a week in addition to cooking with it.

Farmed Salmon: Is it Good for You?
Most salmon is a great source of omega-3 fatty acids. However, the salmon bought from supermarkets is farm raised. They are hatched in plastic trays, crowded into unsanitary underwater cages, fattened with soybean pellets, injected with antibiotics, pesticides, and synthetic dye to give them a deceptive-looking pink color, without which their flesh will be pale gray and unappetizing. The pink dye contains *canthax anthin* that had been banned for human use. Compared to wild salmon, farmed salmon are fatter, they contain two thirds less of the omega-3 fatty acids, and they contain much higher levels of cancer-causing PCBs, dioxins, and more antibiotic residues than eggs, meats, or any other farm-raised animal products. Farmed salmon have high levels of inflammatory messengers while wild salmon have relatively less level of. These inflammatory messengers are implicated in wide varieties of chronic inflammatory diseases like hepatitis. This shift

from wild sea fishing to aquaculture was due to over-fishing and industrial development

Modern Farming

The meats of sedentary domesticated animals have more fats than those in the wild (Vanderhaeghe and Karst, 2004). Wild game that consumes wild plants have very little saturated fat and high essential fatty acids contents when compared with domesticated animals. When animals are domesticated, they are fed with processed foods and put in controlled environments that affect their emotional, physical, and psychological health. The devitalized foods and physical containments impact their immunity to microbial diseases. Domesticated animals are fed growth enhances and feed additives to make them grow and gain weight faster. In the U.S., diary cows are injected with recombinant bovine growth hormones (rBGH), a genetically-engineered hormone used to increase milk production. These hormones leave residues in meat and milk, which can disrupt the natural endocrine equilibrium (hormone balance) in the human body. These have harmful consequences like immunotoxicity, developmental effects, genotoxicity, early puberty, and carcinogenicity. When manure is excreted, these hormones contaminate surface and ground water and harm local and aquatic ecosystems.

"Success seems to be largely a matter of hanging on after others have let go."

William Feather

Conventional agricultural practices use poisonous fertilizers, insecticides, and pesticides derived from petrochemical sources to kill infestations, instead of re-materializing the soil to rectify deficiencies. When humans consume these deficient plants, corresponding deficiencies occur in them. The symptomatic alleviation of infestations with chemicals is a business decision that guarantees repeated use. Traditional agricultural practice encourages low-cost re-mineralization of the soil to address the "cause behind the cause" of the infestations, and strengthens plant immunity to diseases.

The same symptoms that are suppressed with petrochemical-based fungicides are similarly suppressed with drugs in humans. Vegetables produced without rescue chemicals dehydrate with age, while those grown with chemicals spoil after a few days. The soil is the medium for all plant life and the topsoil is the rich, nutrient-laden cover of the Earth's crust from which food crops draw their subsistence. This is where plants are seeded, germinated, sprout, are nurtured, and grown. These plants serve as foods for animals from the highest and lowest end of the food chain. When soil fertility is reduced, there is less life in the soil and the water ecosystem is deprived. Artificial fertilizers cannot be integrated into plant and soil life as bio-organic chemicals. Fertilizers are acid salts that create imbalances by killing microbial life. Pesticides change the genetic structures of humans and animal. Foods grown on depleted soils produce malnourished and diseased bodies (Jensen and Anderson, 1990). Over 300 chemicals are added to our foods and over 10,000 chemical solvents, emulsifiers, and preservatives are used in food processing and storage (Cobb, 2004). These poisons can cause mutations in the body and alter the transmission of genetic (DNA) materials, states Bruyere (1990). Every year in the US.., only 10 percent of the billions of pounds of hazardous wastes produced are disposed of safely without constituting environments hazards (Epstein, Brown and Pope, 1982). It is assumed that most children who have eaten food have half a lifetime's limit of known insecticides and pesticides in their systems by the time they reach their teens (Ausubel, 2000). The government encourages the public to eat five servings of fruits and vegetables a day while failing to note the presence of rescue chemicals contaminating them. The presences of these rescue chemicals contribute to modern immunological diseases.

What is in Beauty Care Products?
In the January 2005 edition of *Alternative Medicine*, Rosemary Carstens indicated that "an estimated 10,000 synthetic chemicals are currently registered for use in the U.S., and fewer than 10 percent of them have been tested for their effects on human health." She believes that an even larger proportion of these chemicals have found their way into cosmetics and personal-care products. Long-term exposure to these chemicals, even in very tiny doses, can be very dangerous. The FDA doesn't regulate the use of these chemicals in cosmetics and beauty aids. Manufacturers are not required to disclose them because of the trade secrets loophole that allows them to be concealed under generic terms such as "fragrance." They are carcinogenic and also disrupt endocrine functions.

Whole Grain Breads versus White Flour Breads: Which is Better? Whole grains are complex carbohydrates that are released slowly in the body. Unrefined whole grains are made whole with three parts, namely the germ, the endosperm, and the bran.

- The germ is that part of the grain that sprouts. It is rich with vitamins which support the plant during sprouting.
- The endosperm is rich in starch and nutrients, which helps the young sprout in its early stages.
- The bran has alkaloids that protect the grain from external influences. It encases the young sprout, is high in fiber, and contains a majority of the minerals in the grain. The protective capabilities of bran are passed on to consumers when consumed whole.

Milling

The milling process affects the nutritional value and quality of flour. Lower-heat methods result in nutritionally-superior flour. Stone-ground flour is milled by a slow process using granite stones, often powered by water, which scatters the bran evenly through the flour and keeps the flour cooler than when ground with steel rollers. Although stone-ground whole wheat flour is still available, most grains today are machine-milled, with superior results. Most of the whole grain flours sold in co-ops are milled by an impact or "hammer mill" that generates almost not heat so the grains do not get scorched.

Refining

After milling, some flours are refined. The refining process strips away the fiber-rich bran and the germ, which contain valuable vitamins and minerals. White flour is refined whole wheat flour. When whole grains are refined (isolated), the germ and the bran are processed out to reduce insect load and increase its shelf life. What is left is only the endosperm, devoid of fiber and nutrients, rich in starch, high in calories, and of no nutritional value. It is simple carbohydrates sold as white bread. This is how wholeness and potency are traded for commercial convenience (Rubin, 2006). Flours labeled as wheat instead of whole wheat are often refined. This sound a lot better than it is. Of the 22 nutrients that are lost in the refining process, only five are added back in the enrichment process.

All I need to know about Flour

Flour, a basic and indispensable food staple, can vary in quality and nutrition depending on the type of grain and the milling process. Baking and cooking with a variety of whole grains adds nutrition and excitement to your meals.

Types of Wheat Flour

Flours made from wheat are the most common. Wheat contains the most gluten. Gluten is a protein. Flours with more gluten make better breads.

- *All-purpose flour* is a blend of whole wheat bread flour and whole pastry flour. This makes a good choice for any of your baking needs.
- *Durum flour* is ground from durum wheat, the hardiest wheat grown. Semolina is refined durum flour. It is the flour commonly used for making pasta. The bran and germ have been removed by an air-sifting process, giving semolina pasta its characteristic light color.
- *Gluten flour* is made from hardy wheat that has been treated to remove some of its starch and concentrate its protein. Gluten flour contains at least 70 percent pure gluten. It can be added to low-gluten flours to lighten the bread. It is also used to make seitan (wheat meat). This is highly refined flour and should be used sparingly to improve bread-rising qualities.
- *Graham flour,* named after Sylvester Graham, an early crusader against commercial white bread, is coarse-ground, whole wheat flour. Used alone, it produces heavy, compact, dark bread.
- *Unbleached white flour* is highly refined. Although it has not been bleached, most of the nutrients have been removed during the refining process. Unbleached white flour is popular because of its versatility. It can be used for breads, pastries, cookies, or cakes. To enhance the nutritional quality, substitute part of the white flour with whole wheat flour.
- *Whole Wheat Bread Flour* or hard whole wheat flour is ground from hard red spring wheat berries, and is best for making breads and rolls.

Other Flours

Flours come from many sources including grains, legumes, starchy vegetables, nuts, and carob, but each has its own baking properties and uses.

231

- *Amaranth flour* has minute traces of gluten and combines well with other flours to make smooth textured breads, muffins, pancakes, and cookies. Amaranth is an ancient Aztec food with an impressive amount of protein, fiber, and minerals.
- *Barley flour* adds a nutty, malty flavor to breads or pancakes. Barley is usually used as a whole grain or in malting, but it is also valuable as flour because it gives breads a cake-like texture and pleasant sweetness. It can also be used as a thickener.
- *Brown rice flour* is nuttier and richer tasting than white rice flour and also more nutritious. It is useful for making breads, cakes, muffins, or noodles. Brown rice flour contains no gluten. Keep it refrigerated to prevent spoilage.
- *Buckwheat flour* is full-bodied and earthy flavored, the traditional flour of Russian blintzes, French Brittany crepes, Japanese soba noodles, and of course buckwheat pancakes. Gluten-free buckwheat isn't really a grain, but a member of the rhubarb family.
- *Corn flour*, more finely ground than cornmeal, is cream colored, slightly sweet, and gluten-free. It is not the same as cornstarch, which is used a thickener.
- *Kamut flour* is from a highly-nutritious ancient form of wheat. Some people who are allergic to common wheat may not react to kamut. Use kamut flour for making breads with a slightly nutty flavor.
- *Millet flour*, ground from whole millet, adds a nut-like slightly flavor to wheat breads. It is gluten-free and traditionally used in some African cuisines.
- *Oat flour* is made by grinding oat grains to a fine consistency. Make your own by grinding rolled oats in a food processor or blender. It has only a small amount of gluten, so if you are using it to make bread, add a gluten-containing flour to help it rise.
- *Potato flour* is made from peeled and steamed potatoes that have been dried and ground. It is stark white in color and very fine. Use it to thicken sauces or it can also be used the same way as brown rice flour. Potato flour is suitable for those on a gluten-free diet.
- *Rye flour* produces a loaf with a full-bodied bitter, slightly sour flavor. It does not contain enough gluten protein to rise well by

itself, and the gluten it contains is delicate. Rye loaves should be kneaded gently to avoid breaking the gluten strands.

- *Soy flour and soya flour* are richer in calcium and iron than wheat flour, gluten-free and high in protein. Soy flour is ground from raw soybeans; soya flour is from lightly-toasted soybeans. Both add a slightly sweet, pleasant flavor to bread. Loaves made with soy flour brown quickly.

- *Spelt flour* is from a non-hybridized wheat with a long cultivation history. It works well as a bread flour and has an exceptional protein and fiber profile. Spelt gluten is highly water-soluble so that it is easy to digest. Spelt flour may be a good wheat substitute for some people who are allergic to wheat.

Pasteurization and Radiation Pasteurization often leads to the destruction of the sparks of life—enzymes. Pasteurization also causes chemical changes in food that destroy nutrients and create genetic changes. Demands are placed on the liver and the pancreas to supply enzymes absent from pasteurized foods (Jensen and Anderson, 1990).

Microwave use damages the molecular integrity of food, which causes structural, functional, and immunological changes in the body (Pitchford, 2002). "The British medical journal, *Lancet*, December 9th, 1989 edition states that the microwave oven transforms amino acid L-proline into D-proline. D-proline is a known nervous system, liver, and kidney toxin."

Irradiation with radioactive elements exposes food to radiation from elements like cesium-137 and cobalt-60 to help kill molds, insects, bacteria, molds, and fungi. This procedure also helps extend the shelf life of food. A study conducted by the Ralston Scientific Services for the U.S. Army and the United States Department of Agriculture (USDA) found that mice fed with irradiated chicken died earlier and had a higher incidence of tumors. Foods devoid of these organic catalysts are classified as dead foods. Rather than nourish the body they drain the body (Cobb, 2005).

Cow Milk: Is it Healthy for You?

Humans are the only mammalian species that consumes milk after the weaning period. Cow milk is cow's milk. It is biochemically incompatible with humans. The lactase enzyme in the intestinal tract—the enzyme that breaks down lactose in milk and milk products—is gone by age three in most humans. The inability of the lactase enzymes to act on lactose consumed after the weaning period leads to milk fermentation in the large intestine. "The fermented products are the gas carbon dioxide and lactic acid. This causes water to be drawn into the intestine by osmosis." (Oski, 1996). More gas and water in the intestines produces a sensation of bloating, resulting in belching, gas, and watery diarrhea, says Oski. Milk and diary products have been shown to contain organo-chlorine pesticide residues (Ausubel, 2000). Cow milk contains casein, which is used as an adhesive wood glue. This substance hardens, adheres to the lining of the intestine, and hampers digestion, and the absorption and assimilation of nutrients. The by products of diary and milk products are acidic toxic mucus, which is the storage place for toxins in the body, an environment for viral multiplication.

Every cell in your body is eavesdropping on your thoughts-
Deepak Chopra
Thoughts are things and moods are place."
Ted Andrews

Doctors Health Advisory: I strongly recommend substituting cow milk with soy milk, goat milk, or rice milk

Recommendations for Future

Holistic medicine, which predates orthodox medicine, is currently referred to as complimentary alternative medicine (CAM). Humanity is best served when all medical practices compliment each other. Health care is a big tent that has room for primitive principles and Ivy League concepts. Both can applied for the ultimate good of humans. Scientific research has greatly improved the quality of life and the standard of living for modern humans. Research has been able to link specific diseases to specific nutrient deficiencies, and supervised use of isolated nutrients in a clinical setting can be beneficial to humanity. Pharmaceutical drugs do have their place when used for crises intervention. They are best used when isolated from natural sources instead of synthetic prototypes.

Harris (2006) indicates that for ultimate health, research should be expanded in the following areas.
- Biologically-based medicine. This emphasizes herbal remedies, vitamins, or the use of special diets that are more bio-availabile to the human cells in terminal diseases.
- Body-based medicine. This includes massage therapy or osteopathy, which encompasses the relationships betweens the nervous system, muscles, bones, and organs.
- Mind and body healing. This includes human spirituality, aromatherapy, meditation, and sound therapy.
- Ayurveda. This is an old Indian practice.
- Healing systems that include acupuncture and naturopathy.
- Homeopathy. This is a healing system that uses all-natural plant, animal, or mineral remedies.
- Energy medicine. This healing approach utilizes the auratic fields to access health status and taps into these energy field to influence healing.
- Reiki. This is a Japanese system of health that uses the laying on of hands to move energy around.
- She is of the opinion that alternative medicine is the largest growing sector in the health care industry. This is evidenced by the development of governing bodies surrounding these holistic therapies.

Appendices

Vegetable Oils for Cooking

avocado	for sautéing and salads
canola	high in omega-3, mild flavor, great for cooking, baking, light sautéing, and salads
coconut	Saturated fat 92 percent.
corn	Good for baking and in salads.
grape seed	High in linoleic acid and low in saturated fats; light, nutty taste; good for cooking.
palm kernel	saturated fat 83 percent; used commercially to prevent candy coatings from melting
peanut	monounsaturated, great for frying, baking, and in salads
olive	Monounsaturated, for salads and light sautéing.
safflower	Great as a salad oil, for cooking, or baking; available in regular and high oleic forms.
sesame	Excellent for stir frying and deep frying; toasted sesame oil is a highly concentrated and aromatic oil added to stir fry or cooked dishes.
soybean	Contains omega-3; has a strong flavor; can be used in cooking, baking and salads.
sunflower	Mild flavor; good for most uses except deep frying; available in regular and high oleic forms.
walnut	gourmet cooking oil; great in salad dressings; high in omega-3
wheat germ	supplemental oil; excellent source of vitamin E.

Supplemental and Body Oils

apricot	Use as a body oil.
almond	Use as a body oil.
borage	Comes from the seed of the flowering herb borage; important as a source of gamma linoleuic acid
cod liver	a good source of vitamin A and D and essential omega-3 fatty acids
evening primrose	extracted from primrose seeds; a good source for gamma linolenic acid
flax seed	supplemental oil that is highest in omega-3; buttery flavor; great in salad dressings, on steamed vegetables, and baked potatoes; also known as linseed oil
fish	often derived from salmon, menhaden, cod, and mackerel; an excellent source of omega-3 fatty acids
hemp	rich in essential fatty acids (EFAs); has a pleasant nutty flavor, and can be used internally or applied topically; is not known whether commercially prepared hemp oil will result in failed drug screening tests
wheat germ	an excellent source of vitamin E and rich in naturally occurring antioxidants

Please note many supplement oils are sensitive to heat and light. Keep themrefrigerated in a dark container. Supplemental oils are not for cooking, but can be added to prepared foods.

The Benefits of Soy foods

The evidence that soy can positively impact your health is growing. Soybeans, and the foods made from them, have a unique makeup. They are rich in a group of compounds called *isoflavones*, which may have some good effects on health.

Isoflavones are one type of a larger group of chemicals called phytochemicals (plant chemicals). Phytochemicals are compounds with a wide range of effects on health and they are found only in plant foods, like grains, beans, fruits, vegetables, nuts and seeds. Isoflavones are also sometimes called phyto-estrogens, which translates to "plant estrogens." Although many plants may contain isoflavones, soy has a particularly rich supply. These can help with preventing cancer and other degenerative conditions.

The number of soy foods available these days is staggering. The most common are tofu, tempeh, soy milk and miso. Newer entrants into the product mix include "veggie" meats similar to Canadian bacon or sausage, and a wide range of products that are soy-based, like salad dressings, snack foods, frozen confections, and entrees.

Miso is a rich, salty condiment. To make miso, soybeans and sometimes a grain such as rice are combined with salt and a mold culture called koji, and then aged for one to three years.

"Second Generation" Soy foods: Many of the newer soy food products imitate meat or dairy products. These second generation products, such as soy deli meats and soy cheeses, fill the demand for meat substitutes while also delivering many of the much-sought-after nutritional benefits of soy foods.

Soy Flour and Soya Flour are richer in calcium and iron than wheat flour; they are also gluten-free and high in protein. They increase the nutritional value of goods baked with them. Soy flour is ground from raw soybeans, while soya flour comes from lightly-toasted soybeans. Both add a slightly sweet, pleasant flavor to bread. Loaves made with soy flour brown quickly.

Soy Milk, also known as soy drink or soy beverage, is the rich creamy milk of whole soybeans. With its unique nutty flavor and rich nutrition, soy milk can be used as a beverage or dairy milk substitute. Soy milk is high in B-vitamins and is an excellent source of protein. Most soy milks are fortified with the same vitamins and minerals as regular milk. There may be ingredients like carrageenin or Job's tears in soy milk, which are plant-based thickening agents that give it a texture like cow's milk, or extra nutrients. Soy milk is also used in the production of many second-generation soy foods, such as ice cream, cheeses and yogurt.

Soy Sauce: Look for a naturally-brewed product made from soybeans, rather than a chemical-based, hydrochloric acid extraction, or imitation sauce flavored with corn syrup. Shoyu is a liquid condiment naturally brewed from soybeans and wheat, and has a light flavor used to dress dishes at the end of cooking. Tamari is a naturally brewed shoyu with a much higher amount of soybeans. This gives tamari a stronger, deeper flavor that is best used at the beginning of the cooking process. Some tamaris are wheat-free.

Tempeh is made with cooked soybeans that are split and hulled, cultured, and then compressed into cakes on large trays to ferment for 24 hours. Tempeh maintains all of the fiber of the beans, and gains some digestive benefits from the enzymes created during the fermentation process. It is a generous source of many nutrients, such as calcium, B-vitamins, and iron. It can be fried or baked, and used in salads, tempura, spaghetti sauces, tacos, or kebabs; it marinades well. Tempeh is usually sold in the refrigerated or frozen foods case. Frozen tempeh keeps for several months. Refrigerated tempeh should be used or frozen by its expiration date. As with other fermented products, a little mold on the surface of tempeh is harmless.

Textured Vegetable Protein (TVP) is made from defatted soy flour and sold in dry granular form. When it is rehydrated, it is used in main dishes as a meat substitute.

Tofu is soybean curd that is low in calories and sodium and is cholesterol-free. It can be an excellent source of calcium and is a good source of B-vitamins and iron. A four-ounce serving of tofu contains just six grams of fat and is low in saturated fat. Generally, the softer the tofu, the lower the fat content.

There are two types of tofu: silken and traditional, which comes in soft (good for smoothies and desserts), firm, or extra firm, the latter two being good for grilling, soups and stir frying. Blocks of tofu can be stored in your refrigerator for one week if they are covered with water, or frozen for up to five months. Frozen tofu has a spongy texture that soaks up marinade sauces and is great for frying.

Tempeh Nutritional Information
Nutrients in one serving of tempeh (2.6 ounces)

Calories	180
Protein	16 grams
Fat	8 grams
Carbohydrate	12 grams
Cholesterol	0
Sodium (mg)	10

Tofu Nutritional Information
Nutrients in one serving of tofu (3.2 ounces)

Type of Tofu	Traditional, Firm	Water-Pack Soft	Silken Firm
Calories	110	86	72
Protein (g)	11	9	6
Carbohydrates (g)	3	3	2
Fat (grams)	6	5	2.4
Saturated Fat (g)	1	1	–
Trans Fat (m)	–	–	–
Fiber (g)	1	–	–
Cholesterol	–	–	–
Sodium	5	5	30

Natural Cleaners

There are Alternatives to Toxic Cleaning Solutions

Some of the worst culprits contributing to environmental pollution are found right under our noses. Petroleum-based household cleaners can contribute to air and water pollution during manufacturing and disposal. The potential environmental and health problems that arise from the use of petroleum-based household cleaners often raises concerns among eco-conscious consumers. There are alternatives to petroleum-based cleaners that are safer, cheaper, and just as effective.

Vegetable-based ingredients, containing acetic or citric acids, have been used successfully for centuries and are based on renewable resources. They also bio-degrade quickly and are gentle on the environment.

In addition, consider using safe concentrated cleaning products. You usually need a fraction of the amount you would with other products. Seek out bulk packaging that is environmentally sound and cost effective.

The Label Reader's Guide to Toxic Cleaning Product Ingredients

Ammonia is toxic when inhaled as concentrated vapors, and is considered a hazardous waste. Ammonia is found in all-purpose cleaners, glass cleaners, laundry detergents, and metal polishes.

Chlorinated cleaners can be especially toxic. Some contain dioxins, a known carcinogen that can build up in the food chain, is stored in fat, and is believed to affect the endocrine system. Chlorinated materials are used in bleach, dishwasher detergents, and toilet bowl cleaners.

Glycol ether is a central nervous system depressant and can poison the kidneys and liver. It is often found in all-purpose cleaners and some laundry detergents.

Oxalic Acid is caustic and corrosive to skin and mucous membranes. It is commonly added to cleaners, toilet bowl cleaners, and metal polishes.

Petroleum-based detergents contain neurotoxins and central nervous system depressants. Exotic-sounding chemicals like nonyl phenol and alkyl phenol ethoxylates (APEs) are found in detergents, furniture polish, cosmetics, and household cleaners, and they contain environmental impurities that contribute to pollution.

Phosphates are added to dishwashing and laundry detergents because they act as water softeners. Phosphates are released into the environment through waste water and are not removed by sewage treatment systems. Phosphates can cause algae growth and suffocation of aquatic life.

Sodium Hydroxide or *Lye* is in most oven cleaners. It is a corrosive poison and hazardous waste.

Clean and Green Cleaning Solutions

With a minimum amount of effort, you can easily make your own cleaning products from inexpensive and common household ingredients. Essential oils are an optional addition to homemade cleaning products and many of them, like lavender and tea tree oil, have anti-fungal, antibiotic, and anti-bacterial qualities. Essential oils also help you make a naturally-scented cleaning product if you prefer to add an aroma to your household environment.

Alice's Wonder Spray ™ Use this recipe for sink, tub, toilet, tile and floors. • ¼ cup white vinegar • 2 teaspoons borax • 32 ounces hot water • ¼ cup liquid dish soap (added last) • 20 drops essential oil (optional) Dissolve Borax in hot water (otherwise the spray will be grainy). Add vinegar, borax, and water to a 32 ounce spray bottle. Add the liquid dish soap and essential oil if desired. Shake ingredients to mix.	Scouring Powder • 1 cup baking soda • ¼ cup borax • drops of essential oil (optional) Mix baking soda and borax together in a bowl or plastic tub with optional essential oil. You can also put the powder in a shaker, and shake it onto the surface to be cleaned.

Drains	Glass Cleaner
For slow drains, pour one cup each of baking soda, salt, and vinegar down the drain. Wait 15 minutes and flush drain with boiling water. Pour boiling water down the drain every two weeks to prevent build up.	Add ¼ cup of vinegar to one quart warm water in a spray bottle. Spray window, rub with a clean rag and dry with newspapers.

Natural Sweeteners

Honey

Honey is twice as sweet as white sugar and contains small quantities of minerals and enzymes. Dark honey, such as buckwheat honey, contains even more minerals and has a stronger flavor than a lighter-colored honey like clover.

Even "natural" honey must he heated slightly during processing and strained in order to remove chunks of beeswax and other debris. Beware of mainstream brands of honey which are overheated, finely filtered (which removes most of the bee pollen), and often processed with sugar or corn syrup.

Honey ought to be kept at room temperature as it may crystallize if it gets too cool. If this happens, place container of honey in warm water until it softens.

Note: Honey may contain botulism spores which can be fatal for infants. Honey should not be given to any child under 1 year of age.

Molasses

Blackstrap molasses is a by-product of the sugar-refining process; it is what is left over after white table sugar has been made from the sugar cane. Blackstrap molasses is very high in minerals such as calcium, iron, and potassium.

Barbados molasses is not a by-product of the sugar refining process, but rather is made directly from sugar cane juice which is boiled down to a syrup. It is not quite as high in minerals as blackstrap molasses.

Because of its strong flavor, molasses is used mainly in baking as a flavoring agent as well as a sweetener.

Agave Nectar

An exciting new sweetener is extracted from the core of the agave, a cactus-like plant native to Mexico. About 35 percent sweeter than sugar with 90 percent fruit sugar content, agave nectar absorbs slowly into the body, decreasing the highs and lows associated with sucrose intake. Agave has a delicious sweet, mild flavor.

Maple Syrup

Maple syrup comes from the sap of maple trees which has been boiled down to make a concentrated sweetener. It takes 40 gallons of maple sap to make one gallon of pure maple syrup. Maple syrup is available in two grades: Grade A and Grade B. (Grade C is no longer a separate grade but has been incorporated in the Grade B classification.) Grade A has a delicate flavor and a light amber color. Grade B is thicker, darker, and has more minerals and a stronger flavor. The grades do not indicate quality of the syrup, only a difference in taste.

Fruit Sweeteners

Fruit sweeteners can be found in products ranging from soft drinks to cereals. The most common fruit sweeteners are apple, white grape, and pear juices, often used in their concentrated form. Look also for fruit sweeteners sold individually, such as Fruit Source® brand sweetener.

Grain Sweeteners

Grain sweeteners are the sweetener of choice of many natural foods enthusiasts, given that they are largely composed of complex carbohydrates and are absorbed slowly by the body. There are two main types of grain sweeteners:

- *Barley malt* is made from sprouted barley and has a rich, malt flavor. It is only half as sweet as white sugar. Beware of brands of barley malt at supermarkets that may have been processed with corn syrup or refined sugar.
- *Brown rice syrup* is made from cooked brown rice and sprouted barley. It has a mild flavor and the highest protein content of any natural sweetener.

Stevia

Stevia rebaudiana, known as sweet herb, is from South America. Sweet glydosides are refined from the leaf into a product known as stevioside. It is 300 times sweeter than sugar. Stevia is non-caloric and does not affect blood glucose levels, so it can be used by people with diabetes or hypoglycemia.

Cane Sweeteners

Sucanat® is a brand name which is an abbreviation for "Sugar Cane Natural." Although it can be used just like white table sugar, Sucanat® is an unrefined sweetener which contains only the dehydrated juice of organically-grown sugar cane. The juice is mechanically extracted, and no chemicals are used during its processing. It contains all the vitamins and minerals sugar cane contains before it is processed into white sugar.

Another unrefined cane sugar, which is lighter in color and milder in taste than Sucanat, is Rapadura. Rapadura is prized for its unique caramel flavor.

Resources
American Liver Foundation
1425 Pompano Avenue
Cedar Grove NJ 01720
201- 256- 2550, 800-GO-LIVER
888-4-HEPUSA, 973-256-2550
www.liverfoundation.org/

Global Hepatitis Support Network
611 Avenue of the Americas, Suite 148
New York, NY 10011
Or
130 Prim Rd, Suite 511
Colchester, VT 08446
802-655-2579

Hepatitis Foundation International
30 Sunrise Terrace
Cedar Grove, NY 07009-1423
800-891-0707, 201-239-1035
www.hefi.org
Email Hfi@intac.com

Latino Organization for liver awareness
888-367-5652, 718-892-8697

Hepatitis B foundation
700 East Butler Avenue
Doylestown PA 18901-2697
215-489-4900
www.hepb.org
Email: info@hepb.org

Hepatitis Education Project
4603 Aurora Avenue North
Seattle, WA 98103-6513
800-2180311
E mail Hep@scn.org

Immunization Action Coalition & the Hepatitis B coalition
1573 Selby Avenue, Suite 234
St.Paul, MN 55104
651-647-9009
Email: admin@immunize.org
www.immunize.org

Immunization Action Coalition &the Hepatitis B Coalition
1573 Selby Avenue, Suite 234
St Paul MN 55104
651-647-9131
Email: admin@immunize.org
www.immunez.org

Latino Organization for Liver Awareness
P.O. Box 842, Throggs Neck Station
Bronx, NY 10465
718-892-8697
888-367-LOLA
Email: mdlola@aol.com
www.lola-national.org

Parents of Kids with Infectious Diseases
P.O. Box 5666
Vancouver, WA 98668
877-55-KIDS
360-695-0293
Email: pkids@pkids.org
www.pkids.org

Hepatitis C Connection
1177 Grant Street, Suite 200
Denver Colorado 80203
303-860-0800, 800-522-HEPC
Email: info@hepc-connection.org
www.hepc-connection.org

Hepatitis C Awareness Project
P.O. Box 41803

Eugene, OR 97404
514-607-6725
Email: hepcaware@aol.com

Hepatitis C Global Foundation
1404 Madison Avenue
Redwood City, CA 94061
650-369-03330
Email:jtranchina@hepcglobal.org
www.hepcglobal.org

Hepatitis C Prison Coalition
P.O. Box 41803
Eugene Oregon 97404
541-607-5725
Email: hepcaware@aol.com
www.hcvprisonnews.org

Hepatitis C Support Project
P.O. Box 427037
San Francisco, CA 94142
415-978-2400
Email: sfhepcat@pacbell.net
www.hcvadvocate.org

Hepatitis Education Project
4603 Aurora Avenue
Seattle, WA 98103-6513
800-218-6923, 206-732-0311
Email: hep@scn.org
www.scn.org/health/hepatitis/index.htm

Center for Disease Control and Prevention
1600 Clifton Road. N.E
Hepatitis Branch, Mail stops G37
Atlanta. GA 30333
888-443-7232, 800-311-3435
Email: dvd1hep@cdc.gov
www.cdc.gov/ncidod/diseases/hepatitis/

Recommended sites for liver disease, detoxification and natural health information, remedies and supplements

For liver diseases, hepatitis B and hepatitis C alternative remedies please visit: www.livershield.net

For natural and alternative remedies for cancer, please visit:www.cancershield.net

For healthy alternatives to overall health problems please visit: www.recoverwithnature.com

Product Selections

You can match the products listed below to the companies listed above. Alternatively, you can go to a nearby health food store and ask for the product s recommended.

- **Milk thistle** Natures sunshine milk thistle, liver lab products, Phytosome milk thistle from Natural factors; phytosome milk thistle from - liver support .com; enzymatic therapy milk thistle.
- **Liver gallbladder formula** – liver lab products, Liver C/S plus from Preventive therapeutic; Liver formula from Organic Health and Beauty; liver formula from Natures sunshine, Liver formula from Natural factors
- **Organic extra virgin olive oil**- Nutriva; Garden of life
- **Whole Super food powdered vegetable formulas**- Vita force from liver lab products, perfect food from Garden of life USA; Miracle greens; Natures sunshine
- **Whole fruits powdered formula**- Radical fruits and fruits of life from Garden of life U.S.
- **Whole food fibers** - Liver lab products, Garden of life
- **Probiotic enzymes**- Natural factors; Preventive therapeutics; Garden of Life USA
- **Digestive enzymes**-Garden of life USA; Enzymatic therapy; Preventive therapeutics; Natural factors
- **Olive leaf extract** -Natural Factors ; Hepatitis C free Pharmacy; Natures sunshine products; Alchemist lab ; Nature's antibiotic Olive leaf Extract distributed by Natural Inc. Island park NY 11588 (Each 700mg capsule contains 500mg of Olive leaf, 150mg of Echinacea and 50mcg of Selenium)
- **Oxymatrine** – Alchemis lab; Hepatitis C free Pharmacy
- **Thymus and liver glandular**: Preventive therapeutics; Alchemis lab; Hepatitis C pharmacy; enzymatic therapy
- **Co-Q10**- Natural Factors; Enzymatic therapy; Natures Sunshine
- **SAMe**- Natural factors; enzymatic therapy; Natures Sunshine
- **Aloe Vera juice**- Lakewood Aloe Vera; Hepatitis C pharmacy
- **Medicinal mushrooms**- Alchemist lab; Natural factors; Hepatitis C pharmacy;

References

Abou-Assi, S., Mihas, A., Gavis, E., Giles, H. et al (2006). Safety of an Immune-
Enhancing Nutrition Supplement in Cirrhotic Patients with History of Encephalopathy. *JPEN,* Journal of Parenteral and Enteral Nutrition 30, 91.

Adodo, A., (2003). The Healing Radiance Of The Soul: *A guide To Holistic Healing.*
Nigeria. Angelex Group

Alan, B.A., Lutz, W., (2000) Life without Bread: *How A Low Carbohydrate Diet Can*
Save Your Life. Illinois. Keats Publishing.

Anderson, A.B. (2004). The Anatomy of Life & Energy In Agriculture. Austin. Acres USA.

Andrews ,T (1989) Simplified Magic. *A Beginners Guide To New Age Qabala*
St Paul . MN. Llewellyn Publications.

Anderson, U.S (1954) Three Magic Words: *The Key To Power, Peace And Plenty*
No Hollywood, CA. Melvin Powers Wilshire Book Company.

Arthur (2006) Holistic Times: *At Risk for Liver Cancer- Something Is Fishy*
Birmingham Al. Clayton College of natural health. 13 (2), 30

Ausubel, K. (2000). When healing Becomes A Crime: *The Amazing Story Of The Hoxsey*
Cancer Clinics And The Return Of Alternative Therapies. Vermont. Healing Art Press.

Avorn, J. (2004). Powerful Medicines: *The Benefits, Risks, And Cost of Prescription*
Drugs. New York. Alfred A. Knopf.

Bailes, F.W (1946) Your Mind Can Heal You
New York. Robert M Mcbridge & Company.

Baker, S.M (2004).Detoxification and Healing: *The Key To Optimal Health*
New York. McGraw-Hill

Balch, J.F. Balch, P.A (2000). Prescription For Nutritional healing: *A practical A To Z*
Reference To Drug Free Remedies Using Vitamins, Minerals, Herbs & Food Supplements. New York. Avery

Baroody, T.A., (2002). Alkalize Or Die: *Superior Health through Proper Alkaline-Acid Balance.* Waynesville. Holographic Health Press.

Barefoot, R.R. (2002). Death By diet*: The Relationship Between nutrient Deficiency And Disease.* Southeastern, PA. Tripod Marketing

Babal, K., Reversing Liver Damage, Nutrition Science News, 2(10), 1997, 508-512.

Bayne, Thomas (2005). Live Protein Therapy in the Management of Liver Disease.
Retrieved 1 April 2006 from: http://www.tldp.com/issue/11 00/protein. htm

Beling, J (1997) Power foods. *Good food, Good Health With Phytochemicals, Natures Own Energy Boosters.* New York. Harper Collins

Bjornsen, K (2006) Phytosterols.
Boulder Co. Alternative Medicine.December, 2006. Issue 92

Bland, J.S., Benum, S .H (1999) The 20-Day Rejuvenation Diet Program: *A younger You In Less Than Three Weeks* Lincolnwood. IL. Keats Publishing

Bolker, J (1998) Writing Your Dissertation In fifteen Minutes A Day. *A guide To Starting, Revising And finishing your Doctoral Thesis.*
New York. Henry Holt And Company, LLC Brown, S.E. (2000) Better Bones, Better Body: *Beyond Estrogen And Calcium.*
Illinois. Keats Publishing.

Brooner Jr., N.H. (2000). Quick Fasting*: How, Why and What To Do*
Atlanta. Century Systems.

Bruyere, R.L. (1994). Wheels Of Light: *Chakras, Auras And The Healing Energy Of The Body.* New York. Fireside

Brundage, A (2002) Going To The sources. *A Guide To Historical Research And Writing.*
Wheeling, Illinois. Harlan Davidson Inc.

Cabot, S (1996) The Liver Cleansing Diet: Love Your Liver And Live Longer
Scottsdale, Az. S.C.N International

Carper, J. (2000). Your Miracle Brain: *Maximizing your Brain Power, Boost Your*
Memory, Lift Your Mood, Improve Your IQ and Creativity And Prevent and
Reverse mental Aging. New York. HarperCollins Books

Carter, J.P. (1992). Racketeering In Medicine: *The Suppression Of Alternatives.*
Norfolk. Hampton Roads Publishing

Carstens, R (2006, January) The Dark Side Of Beauty: *What Cosmetic Companies Don't*
Tell You: Is The Chemical Brewing your Cosmetic Slowly Eroding Your Health?
Alternative Medicine (83) P 67-72

Chen, C., Milbury, P., Lagsley, K. and Blumberg, J. (2005, June). Flavonoids from
Almond Skins Are Bioavailable and Act Synergistically with Vitamins C and E to Enhance Hamster and Human Function? The Journal of Nutrition 135(6), 1366.

Chilton, F.H (2006).Special Report. 30 Diseases. <u>One</u> Solution. *A Universal Antidote*
For Dozens Of Ailments. Emmaus. PA. Prevention

Chilton, F.H (2006). Win The War Within: *The Eating Plan that's clinically proven To*
Fight Inflammation-The Hidden Cause Of Weight Gain And Chronic Disease
USA. Rodale.   Chu, Y-F. and Liu, R.H. (2005). Cranberries inhibit LDL oxidation and induce LDL
receptor expression in hepatocytes. Life Science 77(15), 1892-1901.

Gerber, M., Scali, J., Michaud, A, Durand, M. et al (2000, October). Profiles of healthful
diet and its relationship to biomarkers in a population sample from Mediterranean southern France. Journal of the American Dietetic Association 100(10), 1164.

Geriatrics (1997, July). High daily doses of vitamin E enhance immune response.
Geriatrics 52, 18-20.

Colbin, A. (1998). Food And Our Bones.
New York. Penguin Books

Cobb, B (2005, April) Vegetarian Diet- *Is It Really The Best.*

Sevananda Co-Options. XVII (4), 8

Cobb, B (2004, June) Detoxify And Heal

Sevananda Co-Options. XVI (6), 6-8

Cousins, N., (1979). Anatomy Of An Illness: *How One Man Proved Your Mind Can Cure*

Your Body. Reflections On Healing And Regeneration. New York. Bantam Books

Cohen, R.M. Gish, R.G. & Doner, K. (2001). The Hepatitis C Help Book*: A*

Groundbreaking Treatment Program Combining Western And Eastern Medicine

For Maximum Wellness And Healing: New York. Martin's Press.

Cooperman, T (2006) Beware, One out of every four supplements fails quality testing.

Stamford, Ct. bottom line Health.20 (9), P.1

Cummings, S. Ullman, D (2004) Everybody's guide to homeopathic medicines. *Safe And*

EffectiveRemedies For You And Your Family. New York. Penguin Group

Day, L (2001) Cancer Doesn't Scare Me Anymore (Motion Picture) United States. Rockford Press Inc.

DeCava J.A (Nov, 2005) Essential Nutrition Information. *Of foods & Supplements*

Retrieved August 29th 2005fromwww.home.net/~designed/essential vit min.htm

Diamond, H and Diamond, M. (1987). Fit For Life

New York. New York. Warner Books.

Duffy, W. (1975). Sugar Blues

New York. Warner Books

Duke, J.A (September, 2006) Plant-Based Medicine. *Many Herbs Are Used As Drugs*

Peterborough, NH. Taste Of Life

Dry Cleaning (2005) Environment, Health And Safety Online (EHSO) Retrieved 19th February 2006 from www.ehso.com/ehshome/drycleaningdangers.php

Dyer, W.W (2004) The Power Of Intention: *Learning To Co-create Your world You Way*

Carlsbad, Ca. Hay House Inc

Editorial (winter, 2005) Salmon Is Good For You, Right? *Not* This *Kind* Stamford. Ct. Bottom Line Health, P.3

Ellison, B.J., Duesberg.P.H (1994) Why We Will Never Win The War On AIDS

El Cerrito CA. Inside Story Communications.

Epstein, S., Brown, L and Pope, C (1982) Hazardous Waste In America San Francisco. Sierra Club Books.

Erasmus, U. (1993). Fats That Heal: Fats That Kill: *How Eating The Right Fats And Oils*

Improves energy Levels, Athletic Performance, Fat Loss, Cardiovascular Health, Immune Function, longevity And more. Canada. Alive Books

Everson,G.T., Weinberg, H (2002)Living With Hepatitis B; *A survivor's Guide*

New York. Hatherleigh Press

Ferry, E (June, 2004) Organic And Natural: *A Label Lexicon*

Sevananda Co-Options P 9

Fife, B. (2003) The Healing Miracles Of Coconut Oil.

Colorado Springs. Piccadilly Books.

Filmore, C (1939) Jesus Christ Heals

Unity village, Missouri. Unity Books

Gardner, K (April, 2006) Skin Protection And Vitamin D

Taste Of Life. P60-62

Gilbere, G (2006) What People Need Is Validation

Holistic Times. Clayton College of Natural Health. (13)3, 16

Gilbere, G (2004) I Was Poisoned By My Body...*I Have Got A gut Feeling You Could*

*Be, Too!*Lancaster, OH. Lucky Press Inc

Graves, A (April, 2006) Know Your Water: *Our Most Valuable And Vulnerable*

Resource Taste Of Life. P16-18

Green, J (2000) The Herbal Medicine –Maker's Handbook. *A Home Manual*

Freedom, California. The Crossing Press.

Green, W.F(2002) First Year; Hepatitis B: *A patient-Expert Walks You Through*

Everything You Need to Learn And Do.

New york. Marlowe & company

Haas, E (2000) Staying Health With Dr Elston Haas.Preventing & Treating Colds & Flus

. Retrieved July, 15th, 2006 from www.elsonhaas.com/article_12.html

Harris, W (2006) Take Two Herbal Tonics And Call Me In The Morning: *Holistic*
*Treatments Are Growing As medical Alternatives, Here's What You Need To Know.*New York. Black Enterprise.36 (13), 100-105

Healing Hepatitis Naturally, (2004).
Topanga, CA. Freedon Press

Health On The Net Foundation. *Hepatitis B: Virology And Immunology* (2005, July 26).
Retrieved January 26, 2006 from www.hon.ch/Library/Theme? HepB/virology.html

Hicks, J. Hicks, E (2004) Ask And It Is Given: Learning *To Manifest Your Desires*
Carlsbad, Ca. Hay House Inc

Ho Mae-Wan (2005) The Unholy alliance:
The Ecologist. 27 (4), July August.

Holford, P (1999). The Optimum Nutrition Bible: *The Benefits Of Optimum*
Nutrition. Berkeley. The Crossing Press

Hobbs, C., (2002). Natural Therapy For Your Liver*: Herbs and Other Natural Remedies*
For A healthy Liver. New York. Avery Books.

Jansen, B. And Anderson, M. (1990). Empty Harvest: *Understanding The Link Between*
Our Food, Our Immunity And Our Planet. Garden City Park. Avery Publishing
Group.

Jensen, B. (1999) Dr. Jensen's Guide To Better Bowel Care: *A Complete Program For*
Tissue Cleansing Through Bowel Management. New York. Avery.

Johnson, Mary Ann (2004). Hype and Hope about Foods and Supplements for Healthy
Aging. Geriatrics 28(3), 45.

Karst, k. And Vanderhaeghe, L.R. (2004) Healthy Fats For Life: *Preventing And*
Treating Common Health Problems With Essential Fatty Acids. Canada. John
Wiley and Sons.

Kaido, T., et al. (1998). Perioperative continuous hepatocyte growth factor supply
prevents Postoperative liver failure in rats with liver cirrhosis. Journal of Surgical Research 74(2), 173-178.

Kemp, R.A (1982) Live Youthfully Now
Unity Village. Missouri. Unity books.

Koyfman, Y (2001) Rejuvenate All body systems: *Eight steps to perfect Health*
Norcross, Ga. Koyfman's Center For Health And Rejuvenation, Inc

Kunjufu, J. (2000). Satan, I'M Taking Back My Health
Illinois. African American Images

Lad, V (1984) Ayuverda: *The Science Of Self-Healing*
Santa Fe. New Mexico. Lotus Press.

Lampe, J.W (September1999). American journal Of Clinical Nutrition
.Health Effects Of
Vegetables and Fruit: Assesing Mechanism Of Action Of Action Of Human Experimental Studies. Retrieved 6th November, 2006 from http://ajcn.org/cgi/content/full/70/3/475S. 70(3)475S-490S

Lipski, E. (2000). Digestive Wellness: *Healthy Digestion/Faulty Digestion.*
Illinois. Keats Publishing.

Lipton, B (2005) The Biology of Belief: *Unleashing The Power Of Consciousness,*
Matter & Miracles. Santa Rosa CA. Mountain Of Love/Elite Books.

Leong, W. H. (2003, June). The right vitamin E (the "E" complex).
Total Health 25(3), S22.

Liu, R. H. (2004, December). Potential Synergy of Phytochemicals in Cancer
Prevention: Mechanism of Action1. The Journal of Nutrition 134(12S), 3479. Liu, R.H. and Finley, J. (2005). Potential cell culture models for antioxidant research.
Journal of Agriculture and Food Chemistry 53(10), 4311-4314.

Liu, M, Li, X. Q., Weber, C., Lee, C. Y., Brown, J., and Liu, R. H. (2002). Antioxidant
and antiproliferative activities of raspberries. Journal of Agricture and Food Chemistry 50(10), 2926-2930.

Lyons, G., Stangoulis, J., Graham, R. (2004, June). Exploiting Micronutrient Interaction
to Optimize Biofortification Programs: The Case for Inclusion of Selenium and Iodine.Nutrition Reviews 62(6), 247.

Mathai,K, Smith Ginny(2004) The Cancer Lifeline

Seatle, WA Sasquatch Books

Malkmus, G; Shockey, P and Shockey, S (2006) The Hallelujah Diet

Shippensburg, Pa. Destiny Image

McTaggart, L. (1998). What Doctors Don't tell you: *The Truth About The Dangers Of?*

Modern Medicine. New York. Avon Book.

Mcmillen, S.I (1987). None Of These Diseases*: A Famous Doctors Christian*

Prescription For A Healthier And Happier Life. New Jersey. Spire books.

Mervyn, L (1983) Vitamin E Updated: *New roles For The Vitamin That Preserves The*

Health And Integrity Of Body Cells.

New Canaan. CT Keats Publishing

Mitchell, S (2006) Promoting The Profession

Holistic Times. Clayton college Of Natural Health. Birmingham AL (13)3, 10

Montague, P (1995, March 2) Dry Cleaning: *Is Regulation Necessary?*

Rachael's environment And Health Weekly #431 Retrieved March 11, 2006 from

Www.eject.org/rachael/rehw431.htm

Mowrey, D.B (1986) The Scientific Validation Of Herbal Medicine: *How To Remedy*

And Prevent Disease with Herbs, Vitamins, Minerals And Other Nutrients.

New York. Cormorant Books

Murray Dr (2004, Febuary 9) S-Adenosylmethionine-*A Very Important Product*

Natural Facts. Retrieved September 8, 2006 from www.doctormurray.com/newsletter/2-9-2004.htm

Murray, M. Birdsall ,T. Pizzorno, J. Reilly, P (2002)How To Prevent And Treat Cancer

With Natural Medicine. Ney york Penguin Group.

Murray,M and Pizzorno,T(1998)Encyclopedia of Natural Medicine

Rocklin CA. Prima Publishing.

Myss, C. (1996). Anatomy Of The Spirit: *The Seven Stages Of Power And Healing*

New York. Harmony Books

Odum, L.A (2004, May) Why Detox? *To Protect Your Health, Loose Weight And Slow*

Aging Peterborough, NH. Taste Of Life. Nutritional solutions You Can Trust P21-22

O'shea, T (2005) Sugar: *The Sweet Thief Of Life*
Retrieved January 15th 2005 from www.thedoctorwithin.com

Oski, F.A. (1996). Don't Drink Your Milk: *New Frightening Medical Facts About The*
World's Most Overrated Nutrient. New York. Teach Services Inc

Palmer,M(2004) Dr Melissa Palmer's Guide To Hepatitis & Liver Disease: *What You*
*Need To Know.*New York. Penguin Group

Packer, L and Colman, C (1999) The Antioxidant Miracle. Your Complete Plan For Total Health
And Healing. New York. John Wiley &Sons Inc

Page, L (1999). Detoxification: *All You Need To Know To Recharge, Renew and*
Rejuvenate your Body, Mind and Body. Carmel Valley. Healthy Healing Publications.

Pitchford, Paul. (2002). Healing With Whole Foods: *Essentials Of Nutrition.*
Berkeley. North Atlantic Books.

Pfeiffer, C.C. (1987). Nutrition And Mental Illness. *An Orthomolecular Approach To*
Balancing Body Chemistry. Rochester. Healing Arts press.

Price, W.A. (2004) Nutrition And Physical Degeneration
La Mesa, CA. Price Pottenger.

Primary Cause Of Disease (2005) Fundamentals of longevity
Health perspective.

Reese, M (2005) How well Do Prescription Drugs Work? *The answer May Surprise You*   Sedona. Arizona. Vital Health News. 4 (1), 3

Rosenthal, S.M. (2001). Stopping Cancer At The Source
Canada. Your Health Press

Roselle, G. A (2006) Immune System Weakened By Alcohol
Retrieved. March 27th 2006 from
www.chem-tox.com/immunesystem/alcohol.htm

Rubin, J.S. (2004). Patient Heal Thyself: *A Remarkable Health Program Combining*
Ancient Wisdom with groundbreaking Clinical Research. Topanga. Freedom

Press

Rubin, J.S. (2006, May) Vitamins: Isolates Versus Whole food Nutrition. *The Case For*
Whole Food Nutritional Supplements. Christine's Cleanse Corner.
www.transformyourhealth.com/webnewsletters/may06/nl0506vitamins.html

Saraydarian, H (1973) Cosmos In Man
Cave Creek, AZ. T.S.G Publishing foundation Inc.

Sharma. Mishra, R.A. Meade, J.G. (2002) The Answer To Cancer: *Is Never Giving It A*
*Chance.*New York. Select Books

Schmidt, M.A. Smith, L.H And Sehnert, K.W. (1994). Beyond Antibiotics: *50(or so)*
Ways To boost Immunity And Avoid Antibiotics. Berkeley. North Atlantic Books

Smoking (2006, March 6.) Effects On Your Body
Better Health Channel. Retrieved March 8th 2006 from www.betterhealth.vic.gov.au

Strand, R.D. (2003). Death By Prescription: *The Shocking Truth Behind An*
Overmedicated Nation. Nashville. Thomas Nelson Inc.

Stoll, A.L. (2001). The Omega-3 Connection: *The Groundbreaking Antidepression Diet*
And Brain Program. New York. Fireside.

Starbuck, J (2006) My Natural Cure For Constipation
Stamford, Connecticut. Bottom Line Health. 20(9), p.8

Smartbasics. (1997). Smartbasics *Glossary.*
Retrieved April 18th 2006 from http://www.smartbasic.com/glos.aminos.dir.html . Smythies, J.R (1998). Every Person's Guide To Antioxidants
New Jersey. Rutgers University Press

Timbol, O (2006) Health: Natural Vitamins Or Synthetic
Retrieved March 27th 2006 from www.chiff.com/a/natural-vitamin.htm

Theil, T. and Koff, R. (1999, November). Hepatitis: Know the facts and prevent
hepatitis. The Exceptional Parent 29(11), 78.

Thiel, R.J (2004) Natural Food Complex Nutrition: *Why Are Natural Food Complexes*
Better Than Isolated USP Nutrients? Retrieved April 17th 2006 from www.doctorsresearch.com

Tips, J(2002) The Healing Triad. *Your liver...Your Lifeline*
Austin. Texas. Apple-A-Day-Press
Quillin,P. Quillin,N(2005)Beating Cancer With Nutrition: *Optimal Nutrition Can*
Improve Outcome In Medically-treated Cancer Patients
Carlsbad CA. Nutrition times Press Inc
Veit, R (2004) Research. The Student's Guide To Writing Research Papers.
New York. Pearson Education Inc
Washington, H.A. (2000). Living Healthy With Hepatitis C: *Natural And Conventional*
Approaches To Recover your Quality Of Life. New York. Dell Publishing
Walker, M. (1997). Olive Leaf Extract*: Nature's Antibiotic*
New York. Kessington books
Walker, N.W. (1978). Fresh Vegetable And Fruit Juices*: What's Missing In Your Body*
Arizona. Norwalk press.
Wallach, J.D (August 6, 2005) Black Gene Lies II (Audio)
Men's Fellowship, World Changers Church. Atlanta
Worman, H.J. (1999). The Liver Disorders Source Book
Illinois. Lowell House.
Woodward, A. and Peters, D. (2004, November). Hepatitis. Encyclopedia of Natural
Healing. Retrieved 11 April 2006 from: www.bigchalk.com
Watson and Stockton, S (2006) Essential Cleansing For Perfect Health
Clearwater Fl. Renew Life Press And Information Services
Waters, B (2004). Genetic Breakthroughs are Making Medicines Safe: *The 'Right' Drugs*
Kill 100,000 People A year. Readers Digest, 115-120
Yiamouyiannis,J(1986)Flouride, The Aging Factor. *How To Recognize and Avoid*
TheDevastating Effects Of Fluoride.Delaware Ohio. Health Action Press